PMS

QUESTIONS & ANSWERS

Stephanie DeGraff Bender

❤ **THE BODY PRESS**
A division of
PRICE STERN SLOAN
Los Angeles

Library of Congress Cataloging-in-Publication Data

Bender, Stephanie DeGraff.
  PMS : questions & answers.

  Includes index.
  1. Premenstrual syndrome—Miscellanea.   I. Title.
RG165.B463   1989   618.1'72   88-34215
ISBN 0-89586-815-6

Published by The Body Press
A division of Price Stern Sloan, Inc.
360 North La Cienega Boulevard, Los Angeles, CA 90048
©1989 Stephanie DeGraff Bender.

Notice: The information in this book is true and complete to the
best of our knowledge. The book is intended only as a guide. It
is not intended as a replacement for sound medical advice from
a doctor. Only a doctor can include the variables of an individual's age and past medical history needed for wise medical advice. Final decision about any medical action must be
made by the individual and her doctor. All recommendations
herein are made without guarantees on the part of the author or
the publisher. The author and publisher disclaim all liability in
connection with the use of this information.

10 9 8 7 6 5 4 3 2 1
First Printing

To my partner in life, Bill Bender, and my two
children, Billy and Tim, whose love and
encouragement made this
project possible.

Aknowledgements

I would like to express my appreciation to Bill Bender, Billy Bender, Tim Bender, Judith Wesley Allen, Susan Golant, Rowena Stout, Pam Hopkins, Bruce Fickel, Marla Ahlgrimm, Dave Myers, Joella Good Newberry and all of the people who gave their support and encouragement by contributing their personal questions.

CONTENTS

Introduction

In the last six years I have worked with over 2500 women in the field of PMS. What continues to amaze me is that so many of us have such similar questions. The one that comes to mind first is, "Why do I feel so out of control?" It seems to be standard among PMS women. In fact, it is a question which affects so many areas of our lives that many other questions develop when searching for the answer.

After my first book, "PMS: A Positive Program To Gain Control" was published, many people wrote me with their questions. Since so many people had similar concerns, it seemed logical to address these questions in book form so that other women and men could have access to the answers as well as the knowledge that they were not alone in their situations. This book was written to make positive suggestions for some of the dilemmas that PMS can create.

As a woman who has dealt with her own PMS, I am well aware of how isolating it can be. It makes us feel like we are the only one experiencing those feelings of low self-worth. That way of thinking can keep us from asking for the support and the help that we need.

It is my genuine wish that through reading this book, you will come to realize that you are not alone in your situation and that there are many positive things that you can do to help yourself.

Most importantly, believe in yourself! Trust that what you are feeling is real. Many women have overcome the problem of PMS and have actually learned more about themselves in the process.

Stephanie DeGraff Bender

Foreword

The privilege of writing a foreword to this much needed question and answer book on PMS brings to mind a favorite anecdote. Gertrude Stein, the famed sage and author, is lying on her deathbed in Paris. Her lifelong companion, Alice B. Toklas, is beside her as she seems to finally slip into a quiet death. Just as Alice starts to pull the covers over her companion, Gertrude suddenly sits up. Shocked, Alice blurts out, "Did you find the answer?" The unflappable Stein replied in her famous laconic style, "The answer? I don't even know the question."

Developing questions that lead to the right answers can be very difficult. After ten years of directing and answering thousands of questions from women, I am still amazed at how many improve immediately after obtaining the correct information regarding their disorder.

However, asking the right questions takes a great amount of rigorous experience that can only be developed from direct treatment of PMS patients.

Close to a decade of experience in treating PMS has demonstrated repeatedly that almost 50% of our clinical treatment time is devoted to answering highly relevant questions from today's better informed patients. Therefore, there has long been a desperate need for a book that comprehensively answers the questions about this complex and often perplexing disorder.

Until recently, PMS has been far too often trivialized in the United States. For years, women were shunted away with curt dismissals from their physicians…"It's all in your head!" or simply told to "grin and bear it!" Therefore while 90% of PMS sufferers demonstrate only mild to moderate symptoms that may cause significant but minimal impairment, it is necessary to remember that PMS can often have serious consequences: severe psychological and emotional symptoms as well as debilitating physical problems that can strain relationships, impair the ability to concentrate and work and wreak havoc in the home and in the workplace.

You can't ignore PMS. It won't disappear. PMS is a disorder that worsens with age, stressful lifestyles, poor nutrition as well as certain hormonal body changes. However, our clinical experience clearly demonstrates that PMS is treatable. For most PMS sufferers, simply acquiring an understanding of the disorder and having their questions answered correctly will lead to excellent clinical results.

If you are one of the estimated sixty million American women already suffering from PMS symptoms, it is important that you get the correct information so that you can become responsible for the success of your own treatment.

I do not know of anyone better prepared to lead you comprehensively through the bewildering maze of information surrounding premenstrual syndrome than Stephanie Bender.

Ms. Bender is Director of the PMS Clinic in Boulder, Colorado. She is a nationally known figure in PMS treatment who has already brought her direct clinical experience to the public in her previous book *PMS- A Positive Program To Gain Control.* In addition to her vast expertise in PMS, Ms. Bender is a trained clinical psychologist who is extremely compassionate and sensitive to the problems of the women she treats.

She has a well demonstrated perceptive overview of PMS not only as an isolated hormonally related clinical phenomenon, but as a complex disorder that affects women with numerous physiological, behavioral and social symptoms that need to be understood before they can be treated.

If you are suffering from this disorder, no matter how severe or how minor, use this book precisely as directed, remembering all along the wisdom of Albert Einstein who reminded us, "The important thing is not to stop questioning."

Joseph T. Martorano, M.D.
Medical Director
PMS Medical
New York City

PART I

PMS AND MY BODY

One

WHAT IS PMS?

Q. **What is PMS?**

A. "The world's most common, and probably, the oldest, disease" is the way that one of the world's leading pioneers in the study of PMS, Dr. Katharina Dalton of the University College Hospital in London, describes this cyclic affliction. PMS is a menstrually related physical/psychological disorder that is attributed to hormonal fluctuations that take place in a woman's body. PMS often manifests itself as disturbed mood, sleep and appetite.

Q. **How can I find out if I have PMS? What makes PMS symptoms different from those of other ailments?**

A. The most important criterion in determining whether or not you have PMS is not the symptom itself, rather it is when the symptom occurs. Technically speaking, there are 150 symptoms of PMS. For example, some people may not consider cold sores to be PMS symptoms, but for some women they can be. If a woman finds that she only develops cold sores premenstrually and never during the rest of her cycle, this annoyance is probably a PMS symptom for her. If you are wondering what your symptoms are, chart yourself for a few months and notice when your symptoms appear in relation to your menstrual period.

Q. What do you mean by charting? Can you show me a sample chart?

A. Charting is the daily recording of your most problematic symptoms. Choose two psychological and two physical symptoms to chart (see below). For example, if you have chosen irritability and depression as your psychological symptoms, and breast soreness and headaches as your physical symptoms, you could list them as:

- Irritability
- Depression
- Breast soreness
- Headache

Make thirty-one copies of the chart below—one for each day of the month. Label your chart. Then, preferably each evening, assign a number value from one to ten to the symptoms you've listed. In that way, you can keep track of your numbers when they are highest and consequently, when your symptoms are at their worst. If the high numbers tend to cluster around your menstrual period and disappear subsequently, you are showing a PMS pattern. To further clarify, transfer the numbers for each day to an "on sight chart" monthly so you can review a whole month at a glance.

Q. What should I be looking for when I chart? Specifically, what are the most common PMS symptoms?

A. When evaluating your symptoms, remember that they occur between ovulation and menstruation. The symptoms will cease following the period.

Here is a list of the most frequently cited psychological and physical symptoms:

PSYCHOLOGICAL SYMPTOMS
- Anger
- Loss of control
- Sudden mood swings
- Emotional over-responsiveness
- Unexplained crying
- Irritability
- Anxiety
- Forgetfulness
- Decreased concentration
- Confusion
- Withdrawal
- Sensitivity to rejection
- Depression
- Nightmares
- Suicidal thoughts

PHYSICAL SYMPTOMS
- Bloating
- Weight gain

- Acne
- Dizziness
- Migraine headaches
- Breast tenderness
- Joint and muscle pain
- Backaches
- Changes in sex drive
- Food cravings
- Constipation
- Diarrhea
- Sweating
- Shakiness
- Seizures
- Cold or flu symptoms

Remember that the pattern of symptoms is more important to note than what the symptoms actually are. The following are sample daily and monthly PMS charts. These are adapted from my first book, *PMS: A Positive Program to Gain Control* (The Body Press, 1986).

Q. Besides monthly charting, is there another way to find out if I have PMS?

A. Charting is the most effective, least expensive way to determine if you have PMS. The female endocrine system (which is responsible for your hormones) is very difficult to study because of the sporadic release of hormones into the bloodstream. Blood tests to determine hormone levels would need to be taken daily because of the fluctuations that even "normal" women experience. Therefore, a less expensive, easier, more reliable method to determine if you have PMS is charting. I would stress that charting should be done on a daily basis. We all think that our recall is better than it probably is and daily documentation of symptoms is essential.

Q. **What can I do to recognize whether PMS is causing problems with other areas of my health and well-being?**

A. Chart your symptoms. If the problems with your health and well-being are present to the same degree all month long, you can be reasonably sure that they are not PMS related.

Q. **Doesn't every woman have PMS to a certain degree?**

A. I would not go so far as to say that every woman has PMS. I do think that many women have PMS in varying degrees. If a woman tells me that she feels "blue, grumpy or a little out of sorts" a day before her period, I would suspect she has PMS, but certainly not what I would call significant PMS and therefore, it is probably not interfering with her life.

Q. **How do you determine whether or not PMS is severe?**

A. I call PMS severe when there is physical or emotional damage done to others or oneself during the premenstrual phase.

Q. **Why do these symptoms occur?**

A. There are many different theories regarding the cause of PMS. The most credible is that PMS is a hormonal imbalance resulting from inadequate progesterone during the second half of the menstrual cycle (the luteal phase which begins at ovulation and ends at menstruation) coupled with an excess of the hormone estrogen.

Q. Why does PMS affect so many functions of my body?

A. Since PMS is thought to be caused by a hormonal imbalance, it is reasonably certain that your endocrine system is not functioning correctly. And since all of your organs and organ systems work together one way or another, the imbalance can affect your whole body's functioning. The best example of the wide ranging affects of PMS is cited in the work of Dr. Katharina Dalton, who reported that one of her patients experienced seizures at ovulation and at the onset of the menstrual period. This lead to further investigation that suggested a probable hormonal imbalance which triggered this patient's seizures. After Dr. Dalton worked with the patient and controlled the hormonal imbalance, the seizures disappeared. As I have explained, PMS-related migraine headaches, aching joints, asthma attacks and muscle aches and pains occur only at certain times in the menstrual cycle.

Q. I am unclear on just what roles progesterone and estrogen play in the menstrual cycle.

A. Estrogen stimulates the uterine lining to form

a bed of blood-filled tissue which will receive a fertilized egg. Progesterone helps finish the job of preparing the uterine lining should a pregnancy actually occur. The presence of progesterone is also necessary if implantation of a fertilized egg is to be successful. In the event that no egg is fertilized, both hormonal levels drop. A menstrual period follows.

Q. **What role does progesterone play in PMS?**

A. In a woman who does not have PMS, the progesterone and estrogen levels rise after ovulation, and stay in the correct balance during the luteal phase. In a woman who does have PMS, estrogen will rise, but the progesterone level will not achieve the high level that it should. The resulting discrepancy can result in PMS.

Q. **Since PMS is caused by a hormonal imbalance, isn't there a blood test that checks my progesterone level to tell if I have it?**

A. The endocrine system is one of the most interesting and elusive systems of the body. Hormones are released sporadically, which makes them very difficult to study. Therefore, many hormonal tests are inconclusive and expensive. It is advisable to use more reliable, less expensive ways to check for PMS, such as the daily charting I described earlier in this chapter.

Q. **I've heard that caffeine and salt affect**

breast tenderness during PMS. Why does this happen?

$A.$ Breast soreness is frequently a symptom of PMS. It is also related to your intake of salt and caffeine. Salt depletes the body of potassium. Potassium is responsible for the body's water level. When potassium is insufficient, too much fluid is retained. Therefore, when you eat salty foods, your body retains more fluid. This can manifest itself as breast tenderness. Caffeine has been associated with fibrocystic breast disease. The ingestion of any caffeine will cause breast soreness in many women even when fibrocystic breast disease isn't present.

$Q.$ **How is cyclic constipation connected to PMS?**

$A.$ When you eat food, the digestive enzymes in your mouth and stomach break the food down into chemical units that your body can absorb. From the stomach, your digesting food moves to the small intestine. The job of the small intestine is to absorb the nutrients, such as vitamins and minerals, from the food. The unusable residue moves to the large intestine whose job it is to absorb excess water from the waste product.

When there are no hormonal imbalances, this process takes place as it should. When you have PMS; however, the large intestine can absorb too much water because the body tends to retain fluid. This can result in constipation. Be sure to watch how much salt you eat and make sure that you include enough fiber in you diet to counteract the constipation.

Q. **I seem to be less interested in sex the week before my period. Is this common for all women with PMS? What causes this?**

A. Many women report that their sex drive changes dramatically at different times of their cycle. Not all PMS women report that their desire for sex decreases at the same time each month. For some, it becomes more intense. PMS is a syndrome of extremes, and the symptom of variable sex drive is no exception. When the sex drive is present, it is very strong, and when it is absent, it is really not there. Hormonal fluctuations play a major role in changes in sex drive. In the case of PMS, the fluctuations in sex drive can clearly be connected to hormonal imbalances. Also, many PMS women feel that they need more "space" or distance from their husband or significant other during their premenstrual phase. This certainly would help explain why they don't feel sexual at certain times.

Q. **What is the connection between insomnia and PMS? My insomnia is severe. Often, I can't sleep at all between midnight and 3:00 a.m., I'm alert and feel anxious, but, too tired to even read. During the day, however, I am exhausted and am tempted to take a nap. This situation makes a mess of my job.**

A. Some women report that restless, interrupted sleep is a problem for them during their premenstrual phase. Your sleep cycle may be affected by a neurotransmitter in the brain called serotonin. If serotonin is insufficient, the imbalance can affect the quality of sleep. The level of serotonin is influenced by an amino acid called tryptophan. Tryptophan is found in milk, peanut butter, turkey and other foods. Tryptophan is also available in tablet form at the pharmacy as an over-the-counter preparation. Some people have reported success in controlling their insomnia by using tryptophan to increase their serotonin levels and, ultimately, their quality of sleep.

It is important for you to consider other factors which may be affecting you, such as your pattern of daytime napping. Your body will adapt to a schedule in a relatively short period of time. When a nap is impossible, you may experience tremendous fatigue since you are used to needing the siesta. Even though it may be difficult at first, try to skip your naps, even on weekends. You will then stand a better chance of sleeping at night.

$Q.$ **My doctor keeps telling me there is no connection between my painful periods and PMS. Is this true?**

$A.$ It seems to be the case that the type of menstrual period a woman experiences does not correlate with PMS. For a while, it was suggested that women who suffer from menstrual cramps don't have PMS. Recent research, however, has shown that this is not the case. Just as many women with cramps have PMS as women without them.

$Q.$ **Do women with irregular cycles have worse PMS? I get my period once every two**

months or so. It seems as if my PMS lasts for three weeks before I get some relief when my period arrives! Is this common?

A. Some women with irregular cycles do not have PMS at all. Other women who have PMS and irregular cycles report that they think PMS is worse for them because they never know when to expect their period. In other words, a woman who has a 26-day cycle that occurs like clockwork will have a pretty good idea of how many PMS days she can anticipate. In your case, I suspect that you do not ovulate during the typical ten to fourteen day time span. My guess is that you ovulate later and that causes you to have a much longer cycle. As a result, you may experience PMS from the time that you ovulate until the menses occurs.

Q. **I am a marathon runner. I stopped menstruating for several months when I started training heavily. My periods resumed recently after having been absent for ten months. Now I seem to have symptoms of PMS more severely than ever. My doctor said everything is fine physically. What happened?**

A. Amenorrhea, or absence of menstruation, is the medical term for what you have experienced. It is not unusual for women involved in strenuous physical training to lose their periods temporarily. Your hormonal balance changed enough to stop your menstrual cycle. Even though your periods have resumed, your hormonal levels may not have returned to normal. This can result in PMS symptoms. Try working with self-help measures such as diet, vitamins and exercise (see Chapter Eight) to get your PMS symptoms under control.

Q. My doctor tells me that I have polycystic ovaries. Can that cause PMS?

A. A woman with polycystic ovary disease (PCO) may have excess estrogen in her body because the follicles on her ovaries do not rupture as they should. The excess estrogen has the potential of worsening PMS since the estrogen level is elevated in relation to the progesterone level.

Q. I have endometriosis. Am I more likely to have PMS?

A. There is no correlation between endometriosis and PMS. Some women with endometriosis have PMS and some women with PMS have endometriosis. One of these conditions does not predispose you to the other.

Q. My friend had a tubal ligation and says that her PMS is much worse now. I'm thinking of having this surgery myself. Does this problem happen to other women who have had tubals?

A. Yes, many women report the same result that your friend does. Some studies have suggested that a tubal ligation triggers PMS symptoms. It is suspected that the blood supply to the ovaries and uterus is interrupted by the surgical procedure.

Q. I have fibrocystic breast disease and PMS. Are they related?

A. Even though fibrocystic breast disease does not put you at any higher risk for developing PMS, you may experience more discomfort during your premenstrual phase. The two are related only insofar as the symptoms of the fibrocystic disease become more uncomfortable premenstrually. Conversely, PMS does not put you at higher risk for developing fibrocystic breast disease.

Q. **If I have an ovarian cyst, will this affect PMS?**

A. It could. Ovarian cysts can produce excessive amounts of estrogen. With PMS resulting from a high estrogen level and a low progesterone level, an ovarian cyst can produce the condition.

Q. **Does pelvic inflammatory disease (PID) make me more susceptible to PMS?**

A. Pelvic inflammatory disease could put you at higher risk for PMS. The blood supply to the ovaries could be impaired which would cause them to be less active. Progesterone, the hormone which must be at a high level to prevent PMS, is produced by the ovaries. If the ovaries are impaired, the progesterone level may fall below normal. This could result in PMS.

Q. **Will my fibroid tumors cause PMS?**

A. There seems to be a connection between fibroids and PMS only insofar as they both are affected by hormones. Fibroid tumors grow in the presence of estrogen; however, that would not necessarily connect them with PMS.

Q. How does PMS relate to my other health concerns?

A. It goes back to the "foot bone is connected to the ankle bone" theory. All of your body's systems are interrelated. Since PMS is a hormonal imbalance, it has the potential of affecting many other bodily functions. In some cases, the influence of a hormonal imbalance will be minimal. In other cases, the impact will be pronounced and a cause for concern.

Q. Why do I have headaches each month before my period? Sometimes I have one around the middle of my menstrual cycle?

A. You are describing the two times when headaches are most common in PMS women: during ovulation and right before or at the onset of menstruation. While headaches can be caused by many factors, hormonal imbalances are recognized as a possible cause. You should be charting your headaches to document exactly when they occur. Take your chart with you when you see your health care practitioner to discuss the cycling of your headaches. Be sure you are eating the proper foods and eating frequently during you premenstrual phase (see Chapter Eight) to eliminate the possibility of headaches from hunger.

Q. Is it true that women with chronic disease

such as diabetes mellitus are more likely to suffer from PMS?

A. Women with chronic diseases are not more likely to have PMS. Women with chronic diseases who also have PMS, however, are likely to notice that the symptoms of their condition are more pronounced during the premenstrual phase.

Q. **What about aching joints? Sometimes I think I have arthritis.**

A. Aching joints are reported by some women as PMS symptoms. If your joints ache all month long rather than just during your PMS time, the pain may be due to arthritis. If you do have arthritis, joint pain is likely worsened during your PMS time. But it is unlikely that the achiness will completely disappear during the remainder of your cycle. Keep a chart to see if there is a specific pattern.

Q. **What about allergies? Can PMS affect them?**

A. Your question points out the importance of charting your symptoms. If you notice that your allergy symptoms are present all month long, but that they become more pronounced during your premenstrual phase, it would indicate that they are being affected by your hormonal imbalance.

Q. **I am currently being treated for an eating disorder (anorexia). Over the past year I have lost a great deal of weight. My periods disappeared with my weight. Gradually, the**

weight situation is improving, but I now find myself with premenstrual symptoms. Are eating disorders and PMS related?

A. PMS and eating disorders are related in that severe weight gain or loss can upset your hormonal balance. You have experienced a significant loss and gain within one year. Therefore, it is not surprising that you are dealing with some premenstrual symptoms. Eating disorders can involve issues of personal control. It would be to your advantage to incorporate a PMS component into your anorexia recovery program.

Q. **Do all women have the same PMS symptoms? I experience sore breasts and grouchiness premenstrually, but my mother suffers from migraine headaches. Why do some women have certain symptoms while other women have different ones?**

A. All women do not have the same PMS symptoms. Our bodies are similar and at the same time quite different. Our diets and lifestyles also vary tremendously. A woman who consumes more caffeine and salty foods may experience more breast soreness and abdominal bloating than a woman who doesn't.

Q. **Why is my PMS different every month?**

A. With PMS, variation is the rule. The patterns of PMS can vary from woman to woman and even within the same individual from month to month. In fact, it is misleading to call it premenstrual syndrome because it implies that the symptoms can only occur prior to the period. This is simply not the case with many women.

Some women experience PMS symptoms at ovulation followed by a decrease and then a reappearance just before menstruation begins. Other women experience symptoms during the period itself while still others experience symptoms only before the period begins.

Also, bear in mind that your symptoms may vary in type, severity and duration from month to month. They may stop dramatically with the onset of your period one month, while the next month, they may gradually subside. Charting will help clarify what your patterns will most likely be.

Q. My PMS symptoms are worse about once every four months. Why does this happen?

A. Even though scientists recognize that symptoms and intensity can vary, they are not certain why this occurs. It may be that you eat, sleep and exercise differently from month to month. Also you're not a machine, so your body simply does not operate like clockwork from one month to the next. The variation may also have to do with the differing levels of stress that you are subjected to on a monthly basis. Most likely, it is a combination of all of the above. One thing is clear: most women report variations.

Two

WHY DO I HAVE PMS?

Q. **Can I get PMS if my mother had it? And is my daughter more likely to get PMS if I have it?**

A. At this time there is not enough research available to say with certainty that some women are genetically predisposed to developing PMS. However, many of my patients suspect that their mothers had PMS. In fact, there does seem to be a tendency for a PMS woman's mother or sister(s) to have the problem.

If you have a daughter, educate her about PMS. Be careful not to "set her up" for having PMS by stating that since you have the symptoms she will, too. Have an open discussion with her about what PMS is and how it can be controlled. Then, if she does develop PMS later in life, she is likely to seek help if she needs it.

Q. **Will my PMS be transferred to my sons in some physical way?**

A. Even though it is thought that daughters of women who experience significant PMS may have a greater chance of developing the syndrome, it is doubtful that PMS would affect any male children.

Q. **I have PMS and mood swings as my mother did. Does this mean my daughter will also behave this way?**

A. Many women raise the question of whether or not PMS is a learned behavior. I would seriously consider the possibility if PMS symptoms were strictly psychological. I find it hard to believe, however, that sore breasts, mental fogginess, lack of coordination and cystlike acne can be learned. Physiological predisposition is a more feasible explanation of why PMS seems to run in families.

Q. **If PMS is due to a physiological predisposition, why didn't the syndrome hit our grandmothers like it does us?**

A. Several theories have been suggested. First of all, progesterone is at a much higher level during pregnancy and lactation. Most of our grandmothers had many more pregnancies than we do, and the majority of them breast-fed their babies, so they had much higher levels of progesterone during their reproductive years than we do. If PMS is related to a progesterone deficiency, you can see why this would be significant.

A second theory suggests that our grandmothers had every bit as much PMS as we do, but they saw it as "part of being a woman." As a result, PMS was accepted as a woman's lot in life.

A third theory proposes that our ancestors' diets and activities were much healthier than ours. They consumed less preservatives, salt and sugar and got regular exercise out of necessity. Remember, most of our grandmothers didn't strive to fulfill dual roles the way many of us do. The extra stress of dual roles may account for a higher incident of PMS today.

Q. My mother-in-law has PMS, but I don't. Is it likely that my daughters will get it?

A. Your daughters would be more likely to develop PMS if you or relatives on your side of the family have the condition. Relatives on their father's side would not increase their risk.

Q. When can PMS symptoms appear?

A. PMS symptoms can occur at anytime between puberty and menopause. The most common age for PMS to become problematic, however, is during the thirties. In fact, PMS is sometimes referred to as the "mid-thirties syndrome."

Why is this so? Hormonal fluctuations have the potential to upset the endocrine balance, and for some reason, in some women, the balance is not restored. When these unresolved hormonal fluctuations occur, they can trigger the onset of PMS. We call such events trigger times. As a woman ages, she has more opportunities to experience hormonal fluctuations. A thirty-three-year-old woman has experienced more fluctuations than a twenty-three-year-old by virtue of the fact that she has lived longer.

The most common physical trigger times include:
• pregnancy
• puberty
• taking the pill
• abortion
• miscarriage
• tubal ligation
• hysterectomy

The most common emotional trigger times include:
• death of a close friend or family member
• marriage
• divorce
• remarriage
• relocation

Obviously, these are moments of great stress which can affect your feelings of physical and psychological well-being.

Q. How does stress make my PMS worse?

A. Stress seems to make everything worse! A patient with arthritis, cancer or PMS may notice an increase in symptom intensity when she experiences high stress levels. Stress places an extra strain on all physical and psychological systems. If your body is already hormonally imbalanced, the endocrine system is going to have to work extra hard. This could easily result in a worsening of your symptoms.

Q. **How young was the youngest PMS sufferer you have treated?**

A. The youngest PMS patient I have ever worked with was fourteen years of age. Even though this is an unusually tender age for a woman to experience PMS, it is not impossible for this syndrome to begin with puberty. If you suspect that your daughter has PMS, encourage her to chart her symptoms. Emphasize the importance of proper diet, vitamins and exercise (see Chapter Eight). It can be difficult working with a teenager because adolescence brings with it so many confusing situations. Our bodies are in hormonal flux during that time. (Often hormonal imbalances do straighten themselves out before long.) Add to the changing physiological situation the psychological swings, and I think you will see why adolescence is a difficult process. Be patient if your teenager suspects she has PMS. She needs education, reassurance and some common sense ideas about how she can use self-help measures.

Q. **What can be done to help my child regarding PMS at the onset of menses?**

A. Educating your daughter about PMS is imperative. I would also include in the discussion the fact that not all women experience PMS. If she should develop PMS, however, this condition can provide a wonderful opportunity for the two of you to develop a feeling of camaraderie. What a great built-in support team! Work together to keep the appropriate foods in the house and cooperate in your exercise program.

Q. **Could a sensitive, emotional child be a sign of future PMS?**

A. It is very unlikely that the temperament of a child would be an indication that she would develop PMS in the future. In view of the fact that this is obviously of concern to you, however, why not look into the situation? You might want to check with your daughter's teacher to find out if your child is experiencing problems at school. Also, take into consideration other areas in her life that may be difficult, such as her social activities or home environment.

Q. **How old was the oldest PMS patient you have seen?**

A. Forty-nine years of age.

Q. **I'm a mother of four children. I realize now that I had PMS when I was a teenager. Now my symptoms seem to be more severe and intense. Why is this?**

A. PMS is a progressive syndrome. Many women report that their symptoms seem to intensify and worsen with age. You have experienced several significant hormonal changes in your life brought on by your four pregnancies. As you go through such changes, the chances of a hormonal imbalance increase.

Q. **Does this PMS never end? Will I ever be myself again?**

A. Yes! As a woman who experienced moderate

to severe PMS, I can honestly say that with the proper comprehensive treatment, PMS is very controllable. Your plan needs to correct PMS medically and psychologically. Information about how to regain control by changing some of the behavioral patterns that you adopt during a PMS episode can be found in Chapters Four through Seven.

Q. **I've heard PMS referred to as a progressive syndrome. Can the onset be sudden, such as following the cessation of the birth control pill?**

A. The onset of PMS can be sudden or progressive. Some women report that they think they have always had PMS while others say it started very suddenly following an event similar to the one you describe.

Q. **I'm scared! If this gets worse as I get older, what should I do? I can't stand it now!**

A. PMS gets worse with age if it is ignored. Read through some of the self-help suggestions in Chapter Eight and get started as soon as you can. If those suggestions don't bring about significant alleviation of symptoms, take the next step. Ask you health care practitioner to assist you. Be aware that PMS does not have to get worse if it is addressed adequately.

Q. **How did I live with PMS for so long without knowing that it was a problem?**

A. Many women accept PMS as a fact of life because that is what they have learned. Some women may not realize that they have PMS because the onset is so gradual and insidious. They adapt to the changes and learn coping methods (some of which are unhealthy). Their families develop their own coping mechanisms and, before you know it, everyone is under the assumption that this is the way life is supposed to be.

Life just seems to go on until a crisis occurs. If you slap your child, throw a flower pot or hit your spouse, you may be jolted into the realization that this behavior is not your normal way of dealing with situations. Many times crises motivate us to get PMS under control.

Q. What kind of woman is more likely to suffer from PMS?

A. It doesn't appear that any ethnic groups are more or less likely to develop PMS. I have treated women from all walks of life with PMS and the only common character trait I have discovered is that they are survivors. They possess qualities such as determination, perseverance and strength that have helped them to deal with their situation. Most are determined to conquer PMS. Women in lower socioeconomic groups may have PMS more frequently than others since women who have more financial worries are under stress which can exacerbate PMS symptoms. Certainly, they may not have as much money to spend on purchasing proper foods and vitamins which could affect PMS. On the other hand, women who have no financial concerns can also have problems with the syndrome.

Q. Do overweight women have more PMS than women of average or low weight?

A. Too much fatty tissue can lead to the over-production of estrogen. Because PMS is thought to be caused by a low progesterone level coupled with a high estrogen level, it is possible that over-weight women have a greater tendency to suffer from PMS than women of average or low weight. A vicious cycle can develop where the more over-weight you are, the more fatty tissue you have. This can worsen the hormonal imbalance which could cause more severe PMS symptoms.

Q. Do some regional areas have a higher concentration of PMS cases than others and if so, where are they?

A. I have never been aware of any region which has a higher incidence of PMS. I would qualify this by mentioning that countries where the availability of birth control is limited may have a lower in-cidence of PMS. The women in these countries may experience more pregnancies and, therefore, can have higher levels of progesterone during their reproductive years.

Q. Your first book, *PMS: A Positive Program to Gain Control*, includes examples of married women with children. What about single women (unmarried with no partner), single

women with children and lesbians? Do these other groups suffer more or less?

A. There doesn't seem to be a correlation between incidence of PMS and whether or not a woman is married, has children or is homosexual. I have seen patients in all of these categories, and it doesn't appear that one group or another is more or less likely to have PMS.

Q. **Do women with careers report more PMS than those without?**

A. Most of the women I see work outside the home as well as in the home. That means that they have dual roles. Extra responsibility brings with it extra stress and unfortunately a greater possibility of having more problematic PMS symptoms.

Three

PREGNANCY
MENOPAUSE
AND PMS

Q. **Do women have high or low progesterone levels when they are pregnant?**

A. Progesterone is a very important hormone of pregnancy. Therefore, it is at a high level during pregnancy.

Q. **What about pregnancy and its effect on PMS?**

A. When you become pregnant, your body starts to develop the placenta, a network of tissue and blood vessels that sustains the fetus during the nine-month gestation period. By the end of the first three months of pregnancy, the placenta begins producing twenty to thirty times the normal progesterone. If you experience any early discomforts of pregnancy (such as nausea, fatigue and so on) during the first trimester, these are likely to disappear once you reach the second trimester. It is also possible for these discomforts to be replaced with a sense of well-being. Typically, a PMS patient says that she "glows" during pregnancy. However, once the child is delivered, the placenta is expelled (as the afterbirth), resulting in a dramatic drop in the progesterone level.

How hormone levels affect PMS following the pregnancy varies from woman to woman. In some cases, PMS symptoms intensify following the pregnancy. In others, they seem to decrease. There is no one pattern for all PMS women. From what I have observed with my patients, as many experience less severe PMS symptoms following a pregnancy as experience more severe PMS.

However, you do need to watch for signs of postpartum depression due to the dramatic drop in progesterone levels following delivery. I'll go into this later in the chapter.

$Q.$ **Is morning sickness worse for PMS women?**

$A.$ The first trimester of pregnancy is usually the time that morning sickness (nausea) is present. There doesn't seem to be a clear correlation between PMS and the severity of morning sickness.

$Q.$ **I never had any problems prior to the birth of my child. Now I do. Does childbearing cause PMS?**

$A.$ You have described a trigger time. (See Chapter Two) For some women, the hormonal change that occurs following delivery triggers PMS symptoms.

Q. **I had PMS symptoms in the first trimester of my pregnancy that included headaches, fatigue and depression. They seemed to disappear about three months into the pregnancy. Why does this happen?**

A. Pregnancy is a very interesting time for PMS women because of the fluctuations in progesterone levels. As soon as you conceive, the fertilized egg travels down the fallopian tube and implants in the uterine lining. When implantation occurs, your body gets the message that a pregnancy is beginning. During the first trimester, the progesterone level is somewhat elevated, but not to the extent that it will be later in the pregnancy. Hence, the PMS symptoms continue during the first trimester. The dramatic surge in progesterone at the beginning of the second trimester is probably what caused your symptoms to disappear.

Q. **I had PMS before my pregnancy. It has been eleven months since I gave birth. I nursed my baby for nine months. The whole time I nursed I had no symptoms. I wonder to what extent the PMS will return?**

A. There is no way of knowing to what extent PMS will redevelop. It is important to note that during the time you were breast-feeding these symptoms were absent. That's because your normal hormonal balance is different when you're lactating. Now that you have discontinued nursing, the balance is changing again. It is common for PMS symptoms to return once lactation ends. In your case, it sounds as if the symptoms are fairly mild. It would be a good idea for you to start self-help measures immediately to keep your symptoms in check. (See Chapter Eight.)

Q. **Would nursing my baby alleviate my PMS?**

A. Nursing your baby will not prevent PMS from occurring after your baby is weaned from the breast. It could, however, decrease your chances of developing postpartum depression. When you nurse, your body increases its production of progesterone. In view of the fact that the drop in hormones immediately after birth can result in a depression, you would minimize the possibility of that happening if you nursed.

Q. **I'm going to have a C-section (a cesarean delivery) and I decided not to nurse because of uterine contractions. I've been told that I will be given a medication to dry up my breast milk. Will that affect the potential of my developing PMS?**

A. It is doubtful that the medication would have any bearing on your developing PMS symptoms. I would strongly recommend, however, that you reconsider your decision not to nurse because of the risk of postpartum depression. Ask your doctor to work with you in providing a mild analgesic during the first few days following delivery to alleviate any discomfort you may have due to uterine contractions when the baby is at the breast. In your case, I think the benefits of nursing outweigh the liabilities.

Q. Why would having an abortion bring on PMS?

A. Your hormonal levels change abruptly even in the first trimester of a pregnancy. A woman who has an abortion goes through three dramatic hormonal changes—from non-pregnancy to pregnancy to non-pregnancy—in a very short period of time. The changes in progesterone levels could result in PMS if not properly balanced following abortion.

Q. I've had several early miscarriages and I also have PMS. Are PMS and miscarriage related?

A. Miscarriage can result from many different factors including problems with the hormonal levels. A woman who habitually miscarries in her first trimester should be observed carefully for a hormonal imbalance. Before the placenta is fully developed and is producing the high levels of progesterone necessary to sustain the pregnancy, the ovaries are called upon to keep the progesterone level up. If your ovaries are unable to maintain this essential hormone at the proper level, the product of the uterus will be spontaneously expelled. Since you already know that you have PMS, it would be advisable to explore the possibility that a low progesterone level is causing your miscarriages.

Q. **Do women with PMS have trouble getting pregnant?**

A. Not all women with PMS have trouble getting pregnant. In some cases though, they do. While there are many reasons for infertility, one of them can be a lack of progesterone during the stage when the fertilized egg is trying to implant in the uterus. If progesterone is inadequate at this point, the fertilized egg will fail to implant. Therefore, no pregnancy will result.

Q. **Would a difficult labor and delivery increase my chances for PMS recurring after delivery?**

A. There doesn't seem to be any correlation between the kind of labor and delivery a woman has and the likelihood of her PMS recurring.

Q. **I swelled up in my seventh month of pregnancy. It seemed like PMS swelling. Are they related? Should I be concerned?**

A. PMS and swelling in the seventh month of pregnancy are not related unless the swelling is due to toxemia. Toxemia is characterized by significant fluid retention and high blood pressure. It is a situation that needs to be brought to the attention of your health care practitioner immediately.

Q. **Toxemia was a problem for me. What is its connection with PMS?**

A. Dr. Katharina Dalton states that 86% of

women who have had toxemic pregnancies develop PMS at some time in life. The reason for this strong correlation is unclear.

Q. **I've been having a terrible time after the birth of my baby. My doctor says it is postpartum depression. He thinks I wanted a boy. I had a girl. I don't believe he's right but whatever this is, it's terrible.**

A. What you are experiencing is indeed terrible. You may have a hormonally influenced depression that is compounded by your dealings with a doctor who attributes your state to a problem which you feel does not exist.

When you experience childbirth, your hormonal level changes dramatically. The progesterone level falls off significantly and can affect your emotions. Some women have "the baby blues." This is fairly minor and does not affect them dramatically—they just feel a little down for a few days. On the other hand, some women have severe depression following childbirth.

Postpartum depression has been characterized as being "all in a woman's head" much like PMS. Fortunately, some doctors recognize that postpartum depression is a serious situation that requires medical attention. Why not find a health care practitioner in your area who is more familiar with postpartum depression than the doctor you are currently working with?

Q. **I brought my baby home last week. I should be happy, but all I do is cry. Everyone**

(including myself) is wondering what is wrong with me. Do I need help?

A. Of course you need help. Your body is working to regain its balance hormonally, and it sounds as if it's having some difficulty. You need some reassurance that what you are experiencing could likely be traced to a physiological problem that can be remedied.

You didn't mention whether or not you are breast-feeding your baby. Breast-feeding does increase the progesterone level somewhat, which helps many women with their postpartum depression. Sometimes when breast-feeding is discontinued, a depression is experienced. If you still exprience depression while breast-feeding or feel depressed now that you've stopped, you would do well to seek medical assistance.

Q. **A few years ago I had an abortion. Following the procedure I was told to watch for heavy bleeding. No one told me to watch out for the depression. I still am confused as to why I was so depressed.**

A. Abortion is a very emotional topic for many people even those health care practitioners who perform them. They may tend to emphasize what could happen to you physically (heavy bleeding) and ignore the issue of what could happen to you psychologically.

For some women, abortion will be an emotional land mine. Indecision and conflicting beliefs can render the procedure an agonizing choice. Depression may follow. For others, the choice is very clear. In both cases, however, depression may have a hormonal component. It is entirely possible that your post-abortion depression was related to a deficiency in progesterone following the termination of the pregnancy.

Q. I have PMS. Should I take the pill?

A. If you have PMS, I recommend that you avoid oral contraceptives. The pill contains progestogen, a synthetic form of progesterone. Progestogen and progesterone are not the same substance. The synthetic tends to reduce the natural progesterone in a woman's body by fooling the ovaries into thinking they are already producing adequate progesterone. The result is that they actually make less. In view of the fact that PMS is thought to be caused by too low a progesterone level, lowering it even further is not the answer. In fact, many women with PMS report that their difficulties began when they started taking on oral contraceptive.

Q. Where does the birth control pill really fit into this? My doctor prescribed the pill to help with my symptoms. Shouldn't the birth control pill take away PMS?

A. Many doctors erroneously prescribe birth control pills to control PMS. Oral contraceptives prevent ovulation and PMS symptoms begin at ovulation. These doctors believe that by suppressing ovulation they are also suppressing the cause of PMS. They overlook the fact that the estrogen level rises whether or not you are on the pill. If the progesterone level does not respond accordingly, there will be a discrepancy in the ratio between the two hormones. This imbalance can result in PMS.

$Q.$ **I have felt significantly more in control since I stopped taking the birth control pill. With the pill out of my life, I find that my bad moods more often correspond to an actual issue or event, rather than having no explanation.**

$A.$ Many women with PMS don't tolerate the birth control pill well. Most importantly, you were able to see the correlation and get off the pill. It is always reassuring to see that bad moods actually have a reason and that we are accurately perceiving the situation.

$Q.$ **Can I ever use the birth control pill again? I have pretty severe PMS symptoms?**

$A.$ I would never recommend the birth control pill for you again. We know that it exacerbates the symptoms of PMS in many women. Even if you have gotten PMS under control, I wouldn't risk upsetting the hormonal balance again by using the pill.

$Q.$ **If getting on birth control pills can make my PMS worse, would switching to another form of contraception help alleviate my symptoms or have I changed my hormonal balance permanently?**

A. Discontinuing the birth control pill would certainly be a good idea. It will give your body an opportunity to start producing progesterone at adequate levels. In some individuals, simply discontinuing the oral contraceptive pill and using self-help measures for PMS is all that is necessary to control the symptoms. Other women continue to experience PMS symptoms even after going off the birth control pill. It isn't known whether or not the oral contraceptive permanently changes your hormonal balance. Many variables would have to be taken into consideration, such as how long you were on the pill and the type of pill you took.

Q. **My PMS symptoms are as severe at ovulation as they are just before my period begins. Does this happen to anyone besides me?**

A. Yes it does. It can be confusing because many people assume that once PMS symptoms have begun, they will occur right up until menstruation. With many women, the PMS symptoms will be very severe at ovulation only to subside somewhat and then reappear before the period begins. This pattern is fairly common.

Q. **It appears that sometimes my problems begin a day before ovulation. Is this possible?**

A. It is very unlikely that PMS will occur before ovulation. You may, however, be unsure of how to determine exactly when ovulation occurs. Notice if you have an increase in vaginal discharge. It seems a more reliable indicator of ovulation than waiting for the mild cramping discomfort that may or may not occur. If you are still uncertain, you can purchase a kit that pinpoints exactly when you are ovulating. You can also use the less expensive method of taking a basal temperature which will accurately reflect ovulation.

Q. How closely are PMS symptoms related to early menopausal symptoms?

A. PMS and menopause seem to resemble each other quite closely. In fact, many women wonder if they are going through an early menopause when they first identify PMS. That comes as no surprise when you consider that most of us were educated only about the two Ms: menstruation and menopause. When we start correlating our symptoms (psychological and physical) with the menstrual cycle, the natural conclusion is that our state must be connected to menopause with its emotional ups and downs. In view of the fact that the average age of menopause in the United States today is 51.9 years of age, it is unlikely that a woman in her thirties or even early to mid-forties is experiencing menopause. If your mother is still alive, ask her when she went through menopause. If not, you can ask other relatives. This is the best indicator of when you are going to experience it.

Q. Do women with PMS go through menopause earlier than other women?

A. While there are no statistics available, from my experience, there doesn't seem to be a correlation between PMS and the age that a woman experiences menopause.

Q. **Will menopause be hard on me?**

A. There is no information available which suggests that a woman who deals with problematic PMS is going to have a more difficult or easier experience with menopause. I would guess, however, that if you can balance your body hormonally prior to menopause, you would stand a much better chance of experiencing an easier menopause.

Q. **I had PMS all of my reproductive years. Now I'm menopausal and my doctor is suggesting hormone replacement therapy. Will this recreate my PMS problems?**

A. If your doctor is knowledgeable in the field of hormone replacement therapy, there is no reason for your PMS problems to be recreated. As long as estrogen and progesterone are kept in balance, you should be fine.

PART II

PMS AND MY LIFE

Four

PMS AND MY EMOTIONS

Q. Why does my self-esteem get so low?

A. We all need self-esteem. PMS has a way of chipping away at it because of the regularity with which the syndrome occurs. It is hard to feel good about who you are when you spend the good time of your cycle trying to undo what you did during the bad time.

We often feel as if nothing we do makes a difference when we are in the beginning stages of identifying PMS. We may make promises to ourselves that next month will be better only to find that next month is not any better at all. When this occurs on a monthly basis, it can be very defeating. We may view ourselves as ineffective in the family setting and in the workplace.

I stress the importance of rebuilding self-esteem as a part of the recovery process. Try the following exercise called "restructuring" that is outlined in my first book, *PMS: A Positive Program to Gain Control* (The Body Press, 1986).

RESTRUCTURING

Take some time for yourself. Unhook the phone and have someone else watch the children. Think about one or two of the "mushroom cloud" explosions of emotion that you've experienced lately. As you recall them, you will probably be surprised at how clearly you remember the details. Not only do you remember the cause for the explosion, you also recall what television show was playing in the background! You store all of the grim details about how horribly you behaved in your memory bank. Then, whenever you need amunition to use against yourself, all you have to do is tap into the memory bank and you can see how terrible things were.

As you go through this exercise, also remember that you didn't sit up the night before the incident and plan on being impossible. It happened as a result of a physical problem: PMS.

If at this point you were told that you had diabetes instead of PMS and that a low insulin level was responsible for your going into a rage, you would not blame yourself for past behavior. Even though it is not wise to use PMS as an excuse for your behavior, neither is it appropriate to repeatedly blame yourself for incidents that have taken place in the past. In fact, blaming is counterproductive and will continue to devastate your self-esteem.

Instead, you need to recognize that a habit of beating up on yourself can easily develop when you are dealing with PMS. Month after month you are critical of yourself. This habit did not develop overnight, nor will it disappear overnight. You need to learn how to accept what has happened in the course of having PMS and let go of the habit of blaming. By doing this, you can redirect your energy to regaining your battered self-esteem.

Q. **Sometimes, PMS wears me out just trying to cope. I feel as if I'm not making any progress in family matters. I make promises to myself that next month will be better, but I always seem to fail. In short, I feel ineffective.**

A. How can you feel effective when you fail to keep your promise of change every month? Today's pop psychology says that if we can identify something, we can control it. That leads us to believe that all we have to do to control PMS is to recognize that it exists. However, identifying PMS and the patterns that go along with it is only half the picture. The other part is bringing about change through alterations in habits such as diet, exercise, vitamins and behavioral patterns, such as self-abuse. Women with PMS are experts at being abusive with themselves when every promise they made to themselves isn't kept. This is what I call a behavioral pattern. Be patient with yourself in this area and concentrate on developing an effective support system. Recognize that while PMS is controllable, it does take time to accomplish that goal.

Q. If you are depressed about your life, how much worse can PMS make it?

A. Things certainly seem to be much worse during the premenstrual phase. PMS can cause you to lose your perspective. Often, the situation doesn't change, but the way you view it does. This kind of thinking can only deepen your depression.

Q. Sometimes, the very thought that I have PMS causes me to feel depressed.

A. Your feelings are understandable. No one likes to have anything go wrong in his or her body. Now that you have identified that PMS is a problem for you, use the symptom-free time of the cycle to start working on getting the situation under control. It can be a real lift to see results from your efforts. This can ultimately help you overcome your depression.

Q. What are some immediate steps I can take when PMS creeps up on me? I realize that there are plenty of preventative measure, but I'm not sure what to do in the midst of a crying fit.

A. Interrupt what is happening! There are many options: get something good to eat, go for a walk, take a shower or call a friend. These have worked for me and many of my patients. I'm sure that you can come up with some good ideas of your own. Plan in advance. Tell yourself, "When I get into a crying fit, I'm going to go for a walk even if I have to do it crying."

Q. How do I deal with remorse and guilt after the rages?

A. The anger/guilt cycle is prevalent in PMS women. Use the restructuring exercise at the beginning of this chapter to examine the origin of PMS behavior. Remember PMS is a problem which manifests itself psychologically as well as physically. You must restructure some of the past events over which you may have experienced guilt and remorse. Concentrate on this area because these emotions are connected to your self-esteem which can suffer a crippling blow.

Q. Why do I think of suicide during my PMS time?

A. Sometimes the despair and out-of-control feelings which can accompany PMS lead to thoughts of suicide. Whereas some women who have severe PMS may actually attempt suicide, it is more often the case that a woman entertains the idea and then decides not to go ahead with it. I cannot stress strongly enough that you must share these thoughts with someone you trust who can assist you in getting help for your PMS. This may prevent the recurrence of your suicidal feelings.

Q. Can I mentally control this if I just try hard enough?

A. It depends on how severe PMS is for you. If you have a mild case and are using diet, vitamins, exercise and awareness of your situation, you may be able to control your PMS. However, if you approach the moderate level of PMS, I think telling yourself that you can control it by simply thinking about it sets you up for failure. It is similar to telling yourself that even though you have diabetes, tomorrow you'll get better without taking your insulin. Don't try to convince yourself that sheer willpower can control PMS. If you are not successful, you can take this as an indication that you are weak. Such an attitude may eventually affect your self-esteem, especially if this pattern is repeated on a monthly basis.

Q. **Loss of energy is my biggest problem. I'm almost able to talk myself out of the mental anguish, but I feel totally exhausted. What can I do to have more energy?**

A. I'm not sure if the energy drain you describe comes from your attempt to talk yourself out of the mental anguish or from not eating and exercising properly. If your energy drain results from mental gyrations, hang in there! As you become more familiar with PMS, you will gain a sense of control over it, and it will prove less taxing. In any event, you would probably feel more energized if you follow the recommendations for diet and exercise in Chapter Eight.

Q. **As I bring my PMS under more control, I am aware of the positive aspects of my cyclical changes. For example, when my PMS is very bad I am so sad and depressed I absolutely withdraw like a mole into darkness. When I am controlling my PMS, however, I find I am more introverted before my period. Ironically, I wel-**

come this quiet time as an opportunity for introspection.

A. I think the key is "as I bring my PMS under more control." You are indicating that you are more in control of PMS rather than your PMS being in control of you. "Withdrawing like a mole into darkness" doesn't sound like it would be positive for anyone. I do agree that the introversion that you experience prior to menstruation provides time for introspection which can be valuable. Again, it's important to make the distinction between unhealthy, frustrating isolation that can occur when PMS is in control and healthy introspective time when you are in control.

Q. **I have found that focusing on my spiritual life greatly helps my PMS. When I remember who I am in the eternal scheme of things, I can better balance my emotions. My problems seem smaller and in the right perspective.**

A. It sounds as if you derive comfort from your spiritual life with regard to PMS. I would strongly encourage you to use whatever resources are effective for you.

Q. **Is PMS a mental illness?**

A. PMS is NOT a mental illness. It is a hormonal imbalance which means it is a physical problem. However, because PMS manifests itself psychologically and physically, there seems to be a great deal of confusion surrounding what it really is. When symptoms such as irritability and depression are present, it is difficult, at times, not to think of it as a mental illness. The bottom line is that PMS is a physical problem.

Q. **I have lately made a realization concerning PMS. I have assumed that the hormonal imbalance strips away my ability to keep myself under control and that the person I became during my PMS time is the real me. I am comforted to know that my personality is altered by this disorder, that I am not really this way. Do you think that realization is enough?**

A. While you may be comforted by realizing that this disorder alters your personality, getting PMS under control is more important than working on this realization. I have to agree with you that when you are experiencing significant symptoms of PMS, you are not the real you. The real you is the person who is in control.

Q. **I have panic attacks but only right before my period. Could they be a symptom of PMS?**

A. When anything occurs in a pattern, it could be considered a symptom. In a recent *PMS Access Newsletter*, it was reported that the DSM III, a diagnostic manual used in the field of psychology, lists panic disorders as " . . . a separate entity, distinct from other medical or psychological conditions." There are, however, some studies on panic attacks and anxiety disorders that suggest severe, sustained anxiety is not an illness in and of itself, but a symptom or component of another medical disorder. It is being suggested that the panic attack could be a symptom of another medical disorder, which for you may mean that it is a PMS symptom.

Q. Before I found successful treatment for myself, I had lost three jobs. Because of my inability to function physically or emotionally during my premenstrual phase (which was 60% of the time), I remained unemployed for six months after the last job loss. I went through my savings, and my unemployment checks were about to run out. I thought I was going to end up on the street or in a mental institution. I frankly didn't know where I could go with my problem. It's true that PMS is not life-threatening, except in the most severe cases, but it is destructive to the quality of life for so many people. It also has a severe effect on marriages, parenting and job performance. I know it ruined my reputation as a bookkeeper and forced me to start over again at the very bottom in a new field. The jury is still out on whether my marriage will survive. My story must be repeated many times by other women. Isn't PMS at least as serious a problem as some others? Why are we supposed to suffer and not bother anyone with it?

A. We are not supposed to suffer in silence. However, for a long time PMS received so little attention that research was almost nonexistent. Fortunately, that is changing. I'm not suggesting that things are moving by leaps and bounds, but rather that progress is being made. Your story is repeated many times by many other women. The difference is that now more people in the professional community are starting to realize PMS is real and not imagined. PMS is, as you have stated, at least as serious a problem as some others. It is serious enough to affect you and many other women. I would encourage you to seek out a personal and professional support system that will assist you in gaining control over PMS and rebuilding your life.

Q. How can PMS be a physical problem when I'm experiencing so much psychological distress?

A. PMS is a physiological disorder that manifests itself both physically and psychologically. This seems paradoxical to us because we don't often recognize the two working simultaneously. When a woman is experiencing irritability, depression and anxiety on a cyclical basis, she may still view her problems as strictly psychological. The key here is in understanding that the mind and body operate together. If you are experiencing PMS, there is a hormonal imbalance (physiological) that can and does affect you psychologically as well as physically. Think of a woman who is worried that she is pregnant or really wants to be pregnant. Because the mind and body are connected, it is possible for her to delay the onset of her next period from sheer worry. In this situation, the mind affects the body. If the mind affects the hormones, the hormones can also affect the mind. This results in the severe psychological distress you are describing.

Q. **Why are my emotional problems ten times worse during the two weeks of PMS?**

A. When you experience significant PMS, you tend to lose perspective. Mountains really do develop out of molehills. Your problems don't change during your PMS time, but the way you look at them does.

Q. **My doctor put me on tranquilizers for my PMS. Isn't she saying I'm really crazy?**

A. Your physician is treating PMS as they did in the old days. The unspoken message to you is that there is a mental problem since tranquilizers are used for that reason. Your doctor may be unaware of the message she is conveying. It is important for you to discuss this with her. Let her know what your feelings are. As PMS women, it is easy to feel crazy enough on our own. A professional who is reinforcing that idea is not going to benefit us.

Q. **How many women are misdiagnosed and put in mental institutions when they really have PMS?**

A. We have no way of knowing how many women are diagnosed with a mental disorder when, in fact, they have PMS. My experience with patients suggests that it probably happens more than we would like to believe. Manic depression is probably the diagnosis that many PMS women receive when they report that they have experiences which make them feel like Dr. Jekyll and Mr.

Hyde. PMS can closely resemble manic depression with its ups and downs. However, someone who is truly manic depressive does not experience the symptoms on a cyclical basis as a woman with PMS does. Your question points out the need for mental health and medical professionals to familiarize themselves with PMS.

$Q.$ **Do you foresee a day when doctors don't automatically assume that the problems women have are all psychological?**

$A.$ I think this is changing but probably not as rapidly as we would like. The medical and mental health communities were taught for a long time that women had more psychological problems than men. In the field of PMS, the assumption that this is all in a woman's head excused the medical/mental health communities from looking into what was really wrong. This attitude is gradually changing with women's awareness. The medical/mental health communities' consciousness is being raised in many areas of women's health.

$Q.$ **I have one main concern. It's very easy for me to deny that PMS is a real physiological disorder that causes physical, mental and emotional problems just like booze is the last thing to be blamed by an alcoholic. You can spend years and thousands of dollars bouncing around to doctors and therapists. Doctors say you're fine physically and therapists (even those who claim to understand PMS) get confused and frustrated with you when last week** so much progress was made and you were so positive, and this week you are falling apart again. Soon you really believe that you are nuts! You find yourself locked into a self-perpetuating cycle trying to figure out why you are so miserable when the answer is PMS.

A. Denial is something that many PMS women experience. It is even easier to go into denial when the professionals we are dealing with are not helping us identify the real problem. I think the best tool in dealing with your own denial is to document the symptoms for several months. It is hard to deny that a pattern of PMS exists if it is there in black and white. The documentation is also something you can present to your therapist and physician that will further clarify the situation for them. See my discussion in Chapter One on charting.

Q. **I feel crazy and sometimes people treat me like I am. How can I get out of this trap?**

A. The first thing you can do is believe that you are dealing with a difficult physical problem. Trust that what your body is telling you is real; there is something wrong chemically! Realize that most women with significant PMS feel the same way you do. While I don't want to suggest that a "misery loves company" attitude is healthy, I do want you to take a look around at other PMS women. They have felt exactly the same as you. It is a good reality check! There are many suggestions for other things you can do in Chapters Eight, Nine and Ten.

Q. Is PMS like alcoholism?

A. There are many similarities between PMS and alcoholism. First of all, both conditions affect not only the woman who has the problem, but her family as well. It is therefore recommended that you and your family become educated as to how to deal with the situation.

Secondly, PMS does't appear overnight. It takes months and sometimes years for the syndrome to reach a severe enough level for it to be identifiable. Because of the time involved, you and your family may develop dysfunctional ways of coping without realizing it.

Thirdly, society tends to view PMS and alcoholism as something you can control if you set your mind to it. The implication is that both problems only require willpower. As women who have significant PMS will tell you, they wish controlling PMS were that simple. It isn't.

PMS sufferers also tend to use a great deal of denial. When a woman is in the symptom-free time of the month, she may believe that the syndrome wasn't so bad after all. The tendency to forget how significantly PMS affected her and perhaps her family is one way of denying that a problem exists. Alcoholics can experience similar situations.

Q. Why does my craving for alcohol increase during this time?

A. There are two primary reasons for alcohol cravings during PMS. Alcohol is metabolized by the body as sugar. The blood sugar level seems to fluctuate a great deal during the premenstrual phase, so you may crave sugar at this time. This would account for the need on a physiological level.

Secondly, in this society from the time we are old enough to understand, we hear comments such as, "If you've had a bad day, go home, have a drink and relax." That makes alcohol attractive on a psychological level. We know it is a mood altering drug. If you are dealing with PMS, what could be more appealing to you than to change your mood? It is also the case that you may have an altered tolerance to alcohol during the PMS phase. The worst possible time for you to be consuming alcohol is premenstrually.

Q. **Why do I feel so depressed after I have a drink?**

A. Alcohol is a depressant. When alcohol is consumed during the premenstrual phase, it has an even stronger effect than during the non-premenstrual phase. The depressant effect may be exaggerated also.

Q. **When I am premenstrual, what should my limits be with alcohol?**

A. I suggest that you avoid alcohol altogether when you are premenstrual.

Q. **I still haven't given up alcohol completely. I have a beer every night with dinner. Why is it that sometimes one beer can make me feel as if I've had three or four?**

A. You are noticing an altered tolerance to alcohol that many PMS women report. The liver is affected by hormonal imbalances and does not do as good a job of processing alcohol during the premenstrual phase. Therefore, you may feel an exaggerated effect of the alcohol. Try substituting salt-free sparkling water in place of your beer at dinner time.

Q. A glass of wine seems to relax me and take away PMS symptoms for a short time. Yet, I've been told to stay away from it. Why?

A. Wine contains a great deal of sugar. While you may experience a temporary feeling of relaxation from a glass of wine, be aware that you may pay dearly for it as soon as the relaxing effect wears off, and the depressant effect takes over. You probably have notice the "low" experienced when your blood sugar drops. Try relaxing by listening to music, meditating or engaging in some form of exercise instead of using alcohol.

Q. Why doesn't Alcoholics Anonymous recognize PMS among their female members? They blame my PMS symptoms on alcohol abuse.

A. I don't think it would be fair to say that everyone associated with AA ignores the issue of PMS. After researching the area of PMS and alcohol abuse, I would have to agree, however, that there seems to be substantial resistance to the idea that PMS and alcoholism could be even remotely connected.

While we have noted that PMS and alcoholism overlap in some areas, we must also recognize them as two separate entities both of which require treatment. Your support system (for both alcoholism and PMS) should be airtight during your PMS time to ensure extra encouragement and support. You may need to seek out a support system for your PMS that is separate from AA.

$Q.$ **I'm not an alcoholic, but I've got PMS. My kids are becoming withdrawn and acting out the way I used to with my alcoholic mother. It seems that history is repeating itself only now the problem is PMS. I don't want them to have to go through what I did. What would you suggest I do?**

$A.$ It is helpful to think of a family as a dangling mobile. Each family member is a part of that system. When one part is out of balance, the other parts move to restore the equilibrium. Children will change roles in their attempt to restore the balance in your family.

It is imperative that you talk to your children about what is happening to you. They already have sensed that there is a problem even though it doesn't have a name as yet. By addressing the issue openly, they can get accurate information and feel more in control of themselves with regard to the family and what is happening.

$Q.$ **My sister uses drugs to escape PMS. She numbs up and denies that she has a cyclical** problem. She doesn't limit her drugs to alcohol. She uses a prescription drug from her doctor, too. When one doctor gets wise to her, she finds another one. I guess I shouldn't talk. I used valium for a long time. It numbed me, too. I'm in my second year of sobriety. I can't tell you how long I have had PMS because I can't remember the time that I was numb. My question is how many women do this kind of thing with alcohol and valium?

A. There is no way of knowing how many women are using addictive substances to numb themselves to their PMS. As you have already noted, during the time that you were using valium, you didn't remember much and were unable to get help. Unfortunately, many women have experienced or are experiencing the same dilemma.

Your story also points out the need for the professional community to prescribe tranquilizers on a very limited, short-term basis, if at all, in helping women with PMS. There is always the possibility of doctor-hopping to get another prescription. If the professional community uses good judgment in closely monitoring women in crisis, the use of tranquilizers can be kept to a minimum.

The combination of alcohol and tranquilizers increases the effect of both drugs. This game is deadly; there is a great chance of overdose. Most drugs are labeled to warn of the dangers of mixing them with alcohol. You should point this out to your sister during a time when she is not using alcohol and suggest that she seek out help. You can become her advocate by accompanying her to a professional who will help her with her PMS and chemical dependency problems. Keep in mind that she needs your support and understanding more than anything else.

Q. **Will alcohol interfere with the progesterone I'm using for PMS?**

A. It will not interfere with the action of progesterone, but it will sabotage your efforts to control PMS. You will be introducing a substance which causes a sudden rise and fall in blood sugar level. Alcohol will also cause you to feel depressed.

Q. **Will treating my PMS help my alcoholism?**

A. Treating your PMS may help you get a clearer picture of what is going on and assist you in separating the two problems. Certainly, by getting your PMS under control, you will enhance the possibility of avoiding the craving for alcohol. It will also give you the benefit of starting on a program to have more control in your life. This ultimately may help you with your alcoholism.

Q. **Will treating my alcoholism help my PMS?**

A. By treating your alcoholism, you will probably be doing a lot of soul-searching and self-observation. Most likely that process will help you discover if there is a problem with PMS. If you are motivated enough to be dealing with your alcoholism, I would say the chances are good that you will also be motivated to get PMS under control.

Five

PMS AND MY FAMILY

Q. **Should I tell my children I have PMS?**

A. I can't stress enough the importance of including children in some discussion of premenstrual syndrome. They sense that something is wrong anyway, so why not discuss it with them? It takes away the mysterious air that can accompany a family problem. By talking with them you can make them part of the solution rather than part of the problem. This can be accomplished by asking them to join your support system for the next couple of months until the PMS is under control. You will be surprised at how willing and helpful your children can be when you ask for their support.

Q. **How do I explain this to my family?**

A. Start by addressing the issue during the symptom-free time of your cycle. There is no point in discussing anything when you are irritable and depressed or when your words are coming out backwards. Let your family know that you are concerned about what is happening to you and explain what you are doing about it. You might want to have some reading material available for them should they choose to educate themselves. Emphasize that you are dealing with a physical problem that manifests itself both physically and psychologically. Show them how to be supportive. If they see you actively trying to get PMS under control, they are more likely to appreciate the gravity of the situation and pitch in to help.

Q. **My biggest concern is how to get off the roller coaster of uncontrollably high tension that comes every two weeks between ovulation and my period. My family treats me like a psychopath because I can't tolerate any ripples in my life at all. I can't manage anything that doesn't go along smoothly with my schedule. I need solitary confinement two weeks of every month.**

A. Obviously, you have identified the fact that anything out of the ordinary creates problems for you and your family during the premenstrual phase of your cycle. Typically, a woman with significant PMS will report that she and the people around her are noticing the problem. When you have identified that premenstrual behavior is interfering significantly in your personal or professional life, it is time to chart yourself and start self-help measures.

Q. How can I help my family understand that my irritability is not meant to hurt them and that it is brought on by PMS?

A. Try talking to your family members one at a time. Take some time with each person and explain your understanding of PMS. They need to hear that PMS is a difficult syndrome for each individual who has it. Your family must see you actively seeking help for your problem. By their observing your commitment, they are more likely to understand your situation and support you.

Q. How do I explain to my family the types of feelings, emotions and moods I have when I can't even understand them myself?

A. First and foremost, you need to learn about them yourself. I know this is a difficult task, but it can be accomplished. For example, by learning that low self-esteem is a natural by-product of PMS and finding out that PMS patterns of behavior can lead to low self-esteem, you will be better able to remedy the situation. After you have learned about the emotions, moods and feelings that occur with PMS, you will be in a better position to explain them to family members.

Q. My immediate family walks around on eggshells when I go through PMS. I still have not really been able to make them understand this is a physical thing that I am truly trying to deal with. They ask what they can do, and I really don't have the answers.

A. Many women say that during their PMS time

they want their families near them, but they also want them at an arm's length. It is like saying "I want to go swimming, but I don't want to get wet." A frank discussion with family members describing your emotional state during your premenstrual phase is a great place to start. Paradoxically, letting your family know of your conflicting needs at this time will clarify your behavior and their own reactions. Many family members feel that PMS presents a Catch-22 situation. If PMS is creating major problems in the family, I strongly recommend that you use it as a motivation to get the condition under control.

$Q.$ **My family is not very understanding of the PMS symptoms. Short of getting them to read everything I receive about PMS, how do I get them to understand that I cannot help myself?**

$A.$ First of all, I don't think the answer lies in getting your family to understand that you cannot help yourself because in fact you can. I don't mean to imply that it will be easy, but it can be done.

Suggesting that your family read about PMS is an excellent idea. You might want to follow up with a discussion regarding your personal experiences. Most importantly, they need to see you demonstrate your willingness to get help and help yourself.

Try to find support during the symptom-free time of your cycle. Actively involve your family by asking them to assist you in keeping foods high in sugar and salt out of the house temporarily. I told my children that I needed to banish potato chips from the house at least temporarily. They offered to hide the temptation, but I assured them I would find it wherever it lay. We then agreed to a compromise: no potato chips in the house for three months. Even though this may sound trivial, it made my children feel as if they were contributing to my recovery, and it gave me the support I needed. You could also ask your kids to help you exercise by jogging, walking or biking with you.

Q. When the holidays come, I really feel pressured even when I take progesterone. Is there anything I can do to help make it through these stressful times?

A. Holiday time can be high pressure time for anyone, but especially if you are supposed to be watching your diet, taking time for exercise and keeping stress levels low. It is a good idea to plan ahead. If you're thinking about doing holiday baking, look for recipes that are low in sugar. When attending a party, take some of your healthful treats along so that you don't feel deprived when everyone else is indulging.

It is also a good idea to plan a time for yourself to exercise. Even if it is only a fifteen-minute walk (bundle up, if need be) away from the hustle and bustle you will be surprised what a little open space and change of scenery will do for your mental attitude.

Remember that progesterone is only one part of a total program. It is important to keep all aspects in mind. If you seek the support of your family members during this holiday season, they probably will pitch in willingly, and you will all have a happier holiday.

Q. **Why do I deliberately distance myself from my husband and children?**

A. When you have PMS, you may need every last ounce of energy to put one foot ahead of the other. That means you are going to find ways to save energy for yourself. When you interact with other people, you use up energy. By distancing yourself from others, your family included, you save energy. Address this issue with family members so they don't confuse your need for space with rejection.

Q. **I told some of my family that I have had suicidal thoughts when I was premenstrual even though I have never actually attempted suicide. Now, they call me every day. I know their intentions are good, but they are driving me crazy. What do you suggest?**

A. Your family is understandably concerned about you. They are calling to make sure that you are safe. Make a contract with them; promise that you will contact them if you feel at all suicidal. When they get some assurance that you will let them know when you are troubled, they will be able to relax and take their cues from you. It sounds as if you have a caring, concerned family that you can use as a support system. Take advantage of their interest, and ask for help when you need it.

While it is not uncommon for women with moderate to severe PMS to have suicidal thoughts, it is also an indication that your situation needs immediate attention. Don't wait to see if the thoughts return. Get some help immediately!

Q. I feel that stress increases my PMS symptoms. I am a teacher, and the end of the school year is my most critical time. I often feel very put upon because it seems like I'm the one who has to be understanding and keep harmony in the family. Have other women in these situations found solutions or helpful techniques for maintaining a balance while getting their needs met?

A. Many women have been successful in working out solutions for situations similar to yours. You sound like you have already identified the most problematic time of the year in terms of your stress. There is no question that stress can affect you physically. It comes as no surprise, therefore, that PMS can escalate during high stress times. You need to communicate clearly with family members. Inform them that the end of the school year is a more difficult time for you. Ask for their help! You should not be the only one who is making changes in May and June.

One of the functions of your family is to support you in times of high stress. Ask your husband and children to commit to helping out with household chores or running errands that may be too much for you to deal with. Lists are great because they remind everyone about what they agreed to do. If you can approach your family during a nonstressful time to suggest these strategies, you may be pleasantly surprised to find out how willing they are to help. If that isn't the case, think about what you are willing to give up at the end of the school year in terms of a tidy house, dishes always being done or laundry always folded neatly and put away. It is better to let go of some of these expectations, if temporarily, rather than to over-load yourself and create more stress.

Q. Are PMS and child abuse related?

A. The women I work with report a low incidence of actual abuse towards their children. Many of them say, however, that the thought does cross their minds especially when in the throes of a PMS induced rage.

Most women also report that they are very aware of this thought process and have developed effective interventions, like calling a friend, to pre-vent the abuse from occurring. In many cases, our family members, including our children, create our motivation to seek out help for PMS. In working with thousands of women who have moderate to severe PMS, the incidence of child abuse doesn't appear to be any higher than in the general pop-ulation.

Q. I am very scared because I have come close to physically abusing my son. I feel like yanking him around when I get angry with him. Although he is small for his age, he is very strong. It frightens me that I can feel so out of control. One night I knew that unless I just sat with my head in my hands and talked myself out of it, I might hit him. I waited like that for at least half an hour until my husband came home. During times like that I have suicidal thoughts. These thoughts come; they are not planned. They just come. I am from such a

small town and am a marriage and family therapist myself, so I feel as though I have no place to turn. I feel guilty and tell myself that it will never happen again. It does happen again. I am 43 years old and keep wondering just how much longer I must live this way. I tell myself that once the boys are out of school (in five years) everything will get better. I know that it will improve somewhat, but I also know that I get very angry with my husband for dumb little things. Even though the boys will be gone, my husband won't. I feel desperate.

A. There are several issues that need to be addressed. One of them is fear of potentially abusing your son. One is the suicidal feelings you sometimes experience. Another is the guilt. And still another is that you are a professional who doesn't think professionals can have problems themselves.

It always amazes me that we, as PMS women, feel that the potential is there to really lose control and abuse someone. In reality, however, we usually are more in control than we give ourselves credit for. We expend tremendous energy to keep a lid on our explosive feelings, and we manage, in most cases, to hang in there. You demonstrated your ability to remain in control by not hitting your son. You used an intervention that worked. If you believe that this intervention will not be effective for you in the future, set up a system to call your husband or a good friend when you feel the potential of abusing your child.

The problem of the suicidal feelings can be addressed in somewhat the same way. You need to make a connection with another caring human being when you feel like taking your own life. A phone call to a close friend or your husband would be appropriate at such a time. These two problems are what we call crisis situations. When they present themselves, they call for immediate action.

Your feelings of guilt and the unrealistic expectation that you, as a professional, are not supposed to have problems require more long-term consideration. I see PMS women getting very involved in an anger/guilt cycle which I describe in Chapter Four. It is easy to see how you can feel guilty when you promise yourself that next month will be different, and it doesn't turn out that way. It is also important to identify how and why that happens and to use an exercise called "restructuring" to help remedy the situation.

As far as professionals not having the same problems that their clients do, I would ask you if physicians never get ill or dentists never get toothaches. Of course they do! I don't want to sound flippant or downplay the importance of your feeling in this area because at times I share them. I do want to assure you that being a family therapist does not mean that you are immune to dealing with the frailties of your own human condition. It might be a good idea to seek out the help of another professional (maybe someone outside your community) with whom you can work.

Q. **During my non-PMS times I find myself overdoing it with the kids. I guess I'm feeling**

guilty for when I've been so terrible with them. I know it isn't working!

A. You are engaging in overcompensation, a very common activity for PMS women. You are trying to make up for what did or didn't happen during your premenstrual phase. It is confusing for the children and exhausting for you. We hear from the experts that the most important thing we can be as parents is consistent. Of course, PMS doesn't lend itself well to consistency.

You may also tend to lose perspective of yourself as a parent focusing on the negative interactions with your children and overlooking the positive ones. One of my patients demonstrated this. She told me that during one of her "good" times of the month, she decided to make up for lost time with her three children by taking them to the zoo, the museum and out for dinner all in one afternoon! She was overcompensating. Her zeal caught up with her by dinnertime. She screamed at her kids in the restaurant when a malt hit the floor. The resulting guilt feelings overwhelmed her and sabotaged what she set out to do.

This is also a good example of how we develop patterns of zeroing in on the negative interactions and ignoring the positive aspects. My patient overlooked the fact that the zoo and museum had been wonderful experiences for her and her children. It wasn't until the restaurant that the negative event took place. How much better for her if she had been able to appreciate the positive interactions with her children and not chastise herself for a single incident. How much better for her and her family if she had limited their activities to a reasonable number for one day.

Examine yourself for overcompensation. Do you zero in on the negative and ignore the positive? If you find that these situations are occurring for you, work on writing down a plan to carry out with your children for a day's outing and then stick to it. After you have accomplished that, give yourself credit for being a good mother!

Q. **How do I approach my daughter when I see changes in her right before her menstrual period? When I say something, she comes back with, "Just because you have PMS doesn't mean I have it, too." I am concerned because of her intense mood changes.**

A. Mothers and daughters don't always agree. In your case, your daughter may be in denial about her PMS. Or she may not have it, but your own PMS puts you so much on the alert to the situation you suspect something that really isn't there. In any event, it would probably be helpful for both you and your daughter to avoid the subject for a while. If she does have PMS, she must be the one who decides on getting help for herself. In the meantime, you can do your part by keeping healthful foods in the house and making PMS information available. By effectively taking care of your own PMS, you are providing a positive role model for her should she decide at some point in the future that she does have a problem.

Q. **Should I discuss PMS with my sisters, mother and mother-in-law?**

A. That depends on what your comfort level is with them. If you want to share information for the purpose of asking them to support you, keep in mind that they may or may not believe that PMS is real. If they indicate an interest in being supportive, great! If they do not seem very supportive, don't engage in verbal warfare to convince them that PMS exists. If, however, you find them to be fairly skeptical and critical, look elsewhere for support.

Q. I see PMS symptoms in my sister as well as myself. Yet she becomes defensive when I bring up the possibility that she may have it. What would she most likely be able to hear from me?

A. Your sister needs to come to the point of recognition on her own. If she is in a state of denial about PMS, you can talk until you turn blue in the face, and you won't convince her. Don't dwell on the subject. She may be able to hear you if you address PMS in generic terms or talk about your own condition. If, in fact, she does have PMS, some of the information will ring a bell for her eventually.

Q. Four years ago I was in two mental hospitals because of mood swings. I am now a different person from the person that I was then. I found out I had PMS and started effective treatment. It took me a long time to accept the new me. I have reached acceptance, but my mother-in-law can't forgive or forget the difficulty I put my family through. She is so different towards me at times. She has made comments to some people that PMS is a "bunch of baloney." She feels that my eating habits, exercising, vitamins and medical therapy are for the birds. I feel I have come a long way and even though I am not the same person I used to be, I am still a good person. I have tried hard to make her see me as I am now. It gets really discouraging at times, but I plan on being me. What do you suggest I do? She really won't read any of the information I have on PMS.

A. There isn't much you can do about your mother-in-law's attitude. It is unfortunate that she continues to question the reality of the syndrome for you and your effective method of treatment. Avoid the topic whenever you are around her. And don't put yourself down. You have evidence that what you are doing is working. This is what matters at this point. You might also want to ask your husband if he is willing to suggest privately to his mother that she keep her thoughts on this subject to herself.

Q. My mother-in-law seems to feel that PMS is a modern woman's cop-out. Why sure, she felt some of those things noted as symptoms, but, after all, she is a woman and expected that she would feel them. She leaves me with the feeling that PMS is the "yuppie disease" of the year and that medication, like vitamins, is totally worthless. By the way, she's a nurse.

A. Unfortunately, your mother-in-law's feelings are shared by many people who view PMS as "part of being a woman." I would not buy into what she is promoting. It may be better for you not to mention PMS around this woman. With her attitude, why subject yourself to her cynicism? However, it is important to have a support system which you can rely on to reinforce what you need to do for yourself. An additional thought here: you will find many people in the medical and mental health professions who share her views. Just because she is a nurse doesn't mean she is well informed about PMS.

Q. **My mother had symptoms which I now believe to have been PMS related. I feel terrible that I was so insensitive to her problems . Should I tell her?**

A. By all means! We know that many women who experience PMS had mothers who also had the syndrome. As a child, you had no way of knowing what was going on. Don't blame yourself for something you didn't know. However, now would be a wonderful opportunity for you and your mother to communicate. You can become closer if you are willing to let her know how you feel and what your experience with PMS is.

Six

PMS AND MY RELATIONSHIPS WITH MEN

Q. How can my husband and I cope with PMS?

A. The first thing I suggest you both do is educate yourselves. By gathering information about all aspects of PMS, you can get some ideas about how to deal with everything from dietary changes to family dynamics. I don't want to make this sound simplistic; it's not. However, if you and your husband make a united effort, changes are possible. Start with self-help areas that you can work on together, such as exercising and following a proper diet. From there, take a look at how you and your husband interact during your premenstrual phase. Help one another identify the behavior patterns you have developed as individuals and as a couple. If there are children in the family, you should explore PMS issues that affect them also. I am assuming from the way you worded your question that both of you are interested in getting PMS under control. With that kind of support, the chances are good that you will both be successful.

Q. **My emotional sensitivity the week I have PMS causes conflicts between my husband and me. Fortunately, he is patient and we are able to resolve our problems easily. But in an earlier relationship with a very unstable and insecure person, I would find myself in terrible fights with my partner.**

A. As you point out, the way your partner responds to you is very important. It sounds as if your former companion was contributing to the problem as much as you were. Your experience is a good example of how both people in a relationship contribute to its success or failure. It also emphasizes how important a supportive partner is for a woman who has PMS.

Q. **Although my husband is aware of my mood swings during my PMS days, he still questions the reality of the syndrome. What can I tell him?**

A. In many cases, we base reality on what the rest of the world believes. When other people assert that something is real, we tend to accept it as fact. Because so many people in our society question the existence of PMS, it makes it difficult for sufferers of this syndrome, much less their significant others, to believe that it truly exists. The husband of one of my patients said his wife had seen three doctors who all told her that what she was feeling was all in her head. While the husband wanted to be supportive of his wife, he felt confused. I would suggest you show your husband all the information you can find about PMS, and then discuss it with him. Education is the first step in dealing with this problem.

Q. **How do I handle communication with my husband after I have been hyper-sensitive and angry? I would like to be able to keep my emotions under control when we are discussing sensitive issues, but sometimes I just lose it.**

A. You and your husband should discuss your PMS when the waters are calm. You can be much more objective and communicate more clearly at these times and thus get your point across without upsetting either one of you. Call PMS what it actually is: a physical problem that affects you both as an individual and as a partner in a relationship. You might consider letting your husband know that you are aware of the problems that arise when you become emotional and ask him to cooperate by not engaging in battle with you should a situation arise. By heightening your awareness, you increase the possibility of avoiding conflict. If your PMS is as problematic as it sounds, you would benefit from taking steps to control it.

Q. **My biggest problem is that the special man in my life can't understand why I change so during my PMS days. When I try to explain my feelings and fears during those days I only see**

doubt in his eyes. I give up and try to struggle through this time alone.

$A.$ While I understand your reservations, why not take a positive approach and discuss your thoughts with him during your symptom-free time. You can better communicate your concerns when you are not irritable, depressed, weepy or confused. Encourage him to become a part of your support system. This will help you feel less alone.

$Q.$ **My husband says PMS is a case of mind over matter. How can I make him understand?**

$A.$ You might try the approach I frequently use with the partners of my patients. I tell the man to imagine that he has no money or food and his stomach is growling. Upon the first hunger pang he realizes that he should distract his attention from hunger by engaging in some activity that will take his mind off his pain. As the second and third hunger pangs hit, his attempts will be unsuccessful. Eventually, he will have to respond to what his body is telling him. Reacting to his physiological need forces him to find food. It is not a question of mind over matter when there is an absence of food in the body, so why would it be mind over matter with PMS? After all, this is a physiological disorder.

$Q.$ **PMS is destroying my relationship. My life with this man is a roller coaster of good days and bad. He keeps forgiving me, but how long can I expect him to put up with this?**

A. In my opinion, fairness also can mean being reasonable. The question then becomes, "How long is it reasonable for him to put up with this?" I think it is reasonable for him to deal with your situation for several months during which time you are working diligently at getting PMS under control. You did not indicate whether you are actively working on self-help measures or seeking further medical advice or counseling. It is unfair or unreasonable for a partner if the woman is not working on getting gettting her PMS under control. If she is, I think taking responsibility for her PMS several months is a reasonable time period.

Q. Is PMS a life-long disease?

A. With proper care and attention, PMS does not have to be a life-long situation. After PMS symptoms are contained, they usually remain under control with continued attention to living a healthy lifestyle.

Q. The way my husband responds to me during my PMS days is crucial to my well-being. If he takes my complaints seriously once my symptoms begin, it can be the difference between making me or breaking me. Am I alone?

A. I'm sure other women feel this way. My patients certainly do. No woman likes to be invalidated by her husband. To say that PMS symptoms are trivial, unimportant or, worse yet, imagined, does invalidate us. When we feel as if we are being listened to and considered in a sensitive way it helps us regain control of our situation.

Q. **My husband says PMS is causing major problems in our relationship. He says if it weren't for my PMS everything would be fine. However, I have noticed that during my PMS time he seems to almost invite me to fight with him. I usually respond by accepting his invitation, and we end up battling. Any suggestions?**

A. While there is no question that PMS can create problems in relationships, it is important to acknowledge that it takes two to argue. It is doubtful, even without PMS in the picture, that the marriage would be without problems. Examine what may be a developing pattern. It sounds as if your husband may be setting off a minor explosion when he detects any PMS symptoms in order to avoid a major explosion in much the same way that the mountain service sets off a mini-avalanche in order to avoid a major avalanche. That may explain why he invites you to fight. Another word for that behavior is "baiting." When you are premenstrual you are more likely to take the bait. Then it appears that the problem is caused only by you when, in fact, you are both involved. It is extremely important for both of you to take responsibility for your roles in the relationship. You might want to discuss this situation with an objective third party if you and your husband can't resolve it alone.

Q. My husband, I'm sure, is wondering when the changes will stop. Most of the time, I can handle everday conflicts in a reasonable, adult, non-emotional way. During my premenstrual days, those conflicts become unmanageable, and my reactions are warped. Even telling him I'm premenstrul doesn't help. Sometimes the fight is legit, and he becomes confused about the issues. So do I. For some reason I get really angry at myself and him a day or two before my period. Out of the blue, the shouting happens. I think when a true, non-PMS inspired fight happens I lose credibility because he wants to blame the words and emotions on PMS.

A. You are describing a very familiar concern that many PMS women have: their partners question their credibility in non-PMS related disagreements. It is important to realize that arguments occur in every relationship. To chalk it up to PMS every time would be unfair and even disastrous. Then you assume that every disagreement is due to the woman. Responsibility in relationships is a very important issue. Each party needs to accept his or her fair share. The relationship will become crippled, not strengthened, by continually singling out PMS as the villain.

Q. My husband and I recenty had a discussion regarding issues in our personal relationship. I said, "We need to have time to address these issues." He stated, "Well, isn't your period coming up soon? Maybe we should wait."

I'm concerned that he is using my PMS to imply that I'm not capable of having intelligent discussions. My PMS cannot be used as a scapegoat for putting off the need for intelligent and rational dialogue!

A. I agree that using PMS to invalidate you is counterproductive for the relationship. It also diminishes your self-esteem. Inform your husband about how you feel regarding his use of PMS as a scapegoat. You might set up a time which is agreeable for both of you to discuss your personal relationship and how both of you are addressing your PMS. By doing this now, you have a better chance of avoiding the blowup later.

Q. Why is it so difficult to get my otherwise caring spouse involved in helping me with PMS? Perhaps the better question is, how do I get my otherwise caring spouse more positively involved?

A. The normal reaction to someone who is irritable or depressed is to back away. It can be difficult to get your spouse positively involved because his experience with PMS has probably been negative. He may have some reservations about getting involved at all. In fact, he may try to stay away as much as possible. If he doesn't take that course of action, he may try to fight fire with fire by attacking first. In either case, it's negative involvment. The best way to involve your husband positively is to approach him when you are positive. Provide him with information and express your sincere need for support in dealing with this medical problem. It makes a tremendous difference for both of you when you are operating as a unified front.

Q. **As a newly married woman, I had some major fights with my husband. I noticed there was correlation between the fights and the time of my period. For instance, I often felt like I had poison flowing through my veins at that time of the month that made me even more volatile towards my husband. How much of this could be attributed to PMS and how much to the circumstances of my marriage? We have gotten marriage counseling, and our fights have decreased in intensity, but there are still times when I am somewhat aware of PMS symptoms like extreme emotionalism.**

A. One of the most difficult questions to answer is, "What is affecting what?" Many times I see a woman who reports that she doesn't know what is responsible for the problems she is experiencing in her relationship. As newlyweds, there are certain adjustments to be made by both you and your partner. However, when determining the interaction of PMS, I would suggest that you consider what happens during the non-premenstrual phase of your cycle. Do you and your partner generally deal effectively with your problems during that time? If so, you probably will be able to see to what extent PMS is responsible for your problems. Think of your relationship as being represented by a clear glass of water and the PMS as being represented by handful of sand. When you put the sand into the water and stir it up, you get murky water. It is impossible to tell which are the molecules of water and which the grains of sand. When the two problems exist simultaneously, it can be very difficult to separate one from the other. If you are still experiencing PMS symptoms, you would benefit from working to get them under control. Once that is accomplished, you will have more clarity regarding the other issues in the relationship.

Q. **I sometimes get extremely jealous of any attention the man in my life gives other women. I've never seen this listed as a symptom of PMS, but in my case I think it could be. I feel ashamed, therefore, I do not mention it and how often it occurs. With me, jealousy is so bad it severely affects my life.**

A. I guess technically you could say that jealousy is symptom of PMS. Jealousy really reflects insecurity. If you feel good about yourself, you usually feel secure about your relationships. You know that the person with whom you are involved is as fortunate to be involved with you as you are with him. PMS does tend to foster feelings of insecurity and low self-esteem. If you don't feel good about who you are, why would you expect someone in a close relationship to value you?

However, your partner in reality may be very different from your projection. He may truly value you and the relationship and have no thoughts of other women. I would suggest that you keep a diary of your entire month to determine whether these feelings of insecurity are appearing all month long. It may well be that you are not subject to them during your symptom-free time. However, if you find that your jealousy gnaws at you all month long, find a therapist who can assist you in feeling better about who you are.

Q. **My relationship was almost destroyed by my problems partly because of my emotional withdrawl during my depresseed time of the month and partly because of my lack of interest in sex. How long has it taken other people to rebuild their relationships once they're well?**

A. The length of time it takes to rebuild relationships depends on many variables. Since there are two people in a relationship, both of them have to put some energy into rebuilding it. Even though it is recognized that women, not men, have PMS, everyone will react to PMS in his or her own way. Your husband may interpret your withdrawl as rejection and withdraw himself. The same idea applies to your sexual relationship. Keep in mind that both of you need to become educated about the syndrome in order to recover from it. When you realize that withdrawl on the part of the PMS woman is a way for her to save her limited amount of energy, it becomes less of an issue of rejection and more of a medical problem. When both of you are educated about the fact that dramatic changes in libido (sex drive) are often related to hormonal imbalances, lack of sexual interest is less likely to be taken as a personal affront. I can't stress enough that both of you need to be involved in the recovery process much the same as if you were recovering from a chemical dependency.

Q. Does anything positive ever come from PMS in a relationship?

A. Yes! As a mater of fact, when a couple successfully overcomes the problems of PMS, many times their relationship is strengthened. Any time a couple deals with adversity and comes through the ordeal successfully, the love and respect that were there to begin with are enhanced and enriched.

Q. Rebuilding behavior patterns that are positive in our marriage seems to be an issue right now. With so many of the symptoms gone or under control, our reactions and responses are confused. Where do we begin?

A. You are describing a phenomenon that is common when PMS has been present in a relationship. You develop ways of reacting to your PMS, and so does your partner. I call these behavior patterns. After a while you respond automatically. That is because you have been conditioned to expect certain behaviors. It is very much a two way street when couples are involved. Therefore, when the situation changes and PMS symptoms are under control, you may become confused as to how to react to each other. After all, what should your partner do when the irritability he is used to dealing with isn't there any more? On the surface it sounds like a silly question, and we would assume that the answer would be celebrate. However, as human beings we rely on past behaviors. Your situation would best be handled by both of you recognizing that the game plan has changed.

It would be helpful for each of you to make lists of what you experienced and anticipated in the past. Compare your lists to the situation as it now exists. You may find that your lists are similar. It will also help you to focus on what is happening now as well as what you hope to accomplish in the future. It can be a very positive experience for you to go through such an exercise. If you find that you need more help, consider seeing a professional.

Q. Would counseling help my husband and me with his PMS?

A. Counseling is always a good idea. It sounds like you are referring to a behavioral pattern that your husband has developed responsing to your PMS. It is similar to a situation in which a husband deals with his wife's alcoholism. Education and counseling regarding the impact of PMS on couples' dynamics would be the most effective way to deal with the situation you are describing.

Q. Is there a male equivalent of PMS?

A. No one really knows the answer to that question. There is only one male hormone, testosterone. There are at least two female hormones, progesterone and estrogen. Their interaction can result in imbalances. In the case of males, there is no interaction because only one hormone is present. Therefore, it is doubtful that there would be a hormonal imbalance.

Q. **What about my needs (physical and emotional) during my wife's PMS? Am I supposed to just ignore them and concentrate on her?**

A. During the time that your wife is working on getting her PMS under control, it is natural that she will focus on her problem. Think of this focusing as temporary. If you had been diagnosed with a physical problem, she would be temporarily focusing more on you. However, do not ignore your own needs. They are important. At some point in the discussion on what your wife's needs are, it is essential to address yours as well. If you ignore your own needs, anger and resentment are certain to build.

If you feel that you need some "space," I suggest that you let her know. You could say, "I am going jogging for thirty to forty-five minutes." One suggestion is to exchange time so that each of you gets the space you need during this investigative period. It follows that you will each develop a mutual understanding of your respective needs.

Seven

PMS AND
THE WORLD

Q. **Can I have a career and PMS?**

A. You certainly can, but I must add that severe PMS needs to be controlled in order to have a successful career. Many women realize that PMS interferes significantly with their career. That alone is enough to motivate them to take charge of their condition. Getting PMS under control often helps a woman realize how limited she has been and gives her the impetus to advance further in her career.

Q. **I am afraid to commit to long, difficult projects because of PMS. For example, I've been accepted to a fairly prestigious graduate school. Committing to this three-year ordeal means that I will not be able to afford time off for medical reasons. Although I have the ability to succeed in graduate school, I also know**

that PMS can cripple my mind and body to the point where I can't even pick up a pencil, much less study. Because of PMS, I often feel inadequate.

A. Unfortunately, you are suffering from a defeatist mind-set. You tend to generalize that your past experiences with PMS will repeat themselves the rest of your life. While this is understandable, it is important that you reconsider your situation. When PMS is most problematic, you may experience yourself as crippled both mentally and physically. You are also stripped of your self-confidence because you have experienced situations during your PMS times when your judgment proved to be unreliable. You then perceive this PMS state as spilling over into the rest of the month. It all fits together so neatly but dangerously.

It is time for you to see that with proper treatment, you can gain control over PMS so that you don't experience these crippling effects. You can mentally and physically return to a point where you will be only minimally affected. When you start to experience the return to normalcy, you will need to work consciously at taking small risks. Notice your success as you deal with each challenge effectively. During this process, you will be building a foundation upon which you can expand. Eventually, you will see that you are capable of dealing with graduate school. By virtue of the fact that you have been accepted to a graduate school, you must have records that reflect your past accomplishments. Use this as a reality check that proves your capability. There is no reason to stay stuck in the PMS mind-set that implies what you are currently experiencing will continue for the rest of your life. Many women have overcome this kind of thinking and you can, too.

Q. Is PMS becoming an issue in the workplace?

A. Yes, PMS is becoming an issue for the women who have it and the people for whom they work. Given the fact that PMS is a medical disorder, it needs to be addressed by both the employer and the employee. Eventually, even the smallest considerations, such as having juice and decaffeinated coffee available for breaks, will be accomodated.

Q. What can I do about getting my boss to understand PMS?

A. Education is the name of the game. As more is written about PMS, the subject is gaining credibility. I would suggest that you gather information regarding PMS and give it to your boss. You then might offer to discuss the topic once he or she has read the literature to further clarify the situation. By sharing information about PMS from sources other than yourself, you are also validating the reality of the syndrome. If possible, you may want to suggest inviting a guest speaker to discuss the topic with the staff.

Q. How should I tell my boss that I think I have PMS? I'm afraid it will jeopardize my job.

A. Whether or not you tell your boss about your PMS is strictly your decision. If PMS is interfering with your performance at work, obviously you need to be doing something about it. That does not mean that you have to tell your boss that you have PMS. You can simply tell him or her that you are dealing with a medical problem and that it should be cleared up within the next month or two. If you were diagnosed with diabetes, you would also need a few months to balance out diet, exercise and medication. With PMS you are facing a situation that can be controlled effectively if the right measures are taken.

Q. **What can I do to have my place of employment help me during my PMS? I would like to be as productive during my PMS days as my non-PMS days.**

A. Educational programs for management are probably the most effective tool. I encourage companies to have employment assistant programs (EAP) to keep information available about PMS just as they do with programs dealing with chemical dependency. Ideally, it would be great for all concerned if you control your PMS. Then every day of the month can be productive.

Q. **How do I get treatment without my boss thinking I'm irrational?**

A. Many patients worry about this. If your PMS is significant enough to interfere with your work, it is up to you to seek help so that you can get the situation under control. Treatment for PMS should be available with the same confidentiality as with any other medical problem. Therefore, there is no reason for any woman to deny herself treatment.

Q. **Is the divorce rate, number of accidents and job loss rate high among PMS sufferers?**

A. Many of our clients report that PMS played a significant role in all of the situations you have mentioned. Again, it points out the importance of accurate information regarding PMS so that we can control the syndrome rather than having the syndrome control us.

Q. **I have had severe PMS for five years. It started when my doctor took me off birth control pills at age 39. My husband has filed for a divorce, and I will now have to support myself. My symptoms are extremely emotional. On bad days, I'll cry for four to five hours straight. I'm worried that I will not be able to obtain or hold down a job. I was fired from my last job because of an incident that occured during a PMS episode. What do other women do in the workplace to deal with the extreme emotional aspects of PMS?**

A. Many women have had similar experiences. Your PMS sounds fairly extreme. It also sounds like you need help in getting other areas of your life in order. Getting your PMS under control should be the first step you make in going through this difficult time. By taking care of this, other areas, such as work and relationships, will be more manageable for you. Enlist the help of a professional counselor as soon as possible. Dismiss the events in your past work experiences as ancient history and tackle the problem of PMS in your workplace from a new angle. By getting your PMS under control, there is no reason to expect that you will have the same emotional outbursts of the past.

Q. **Does anyone else experience impaired intellectual ability premenstrually? While I was a student, I couldn't keep up with my schoolwork during my PMS days, but I had no problem the rest of the time. Later, when I worked as a bookkeeper, I could not add two two-digit numbers together correctly during my bad times. Also, when speaking, I would go blank on a word in almost every sentence.**

A. Many women report that they become "foggy" mentally during the premenstrual phase. It has been suggested that this may be due to a fluctuation in the blood sugar level. Consider eating on a hypoglycemic diet schedule. That schedule requires you to eat six small meals per day: breakfast, snack, lunch, snack, dinner and evening snack. Naturally, what you eat is as important as when you eat. Be sure that you eliminate caffeine and alcohol, and keep your sugar and salt intake to a minimum. Increasing your intake of fruits, vegetables and complex carbohydrates is a good idea. Getting the proper amount of rest and exercise is very important. Make sure you exercise at least three times per week for a minimum of a half-hour each time. There are a number of self-help suggestions in Chapter Eight that should also help.

$Q.$ **I do most of my work at the office during my good time of the month. That adds up to an exhausting two weeks. Do you have any suggestions?**

$A.$ You are describing a phenomenon shared by many PMS sufferers who work outside the home. You are tempted to get a month's worth of work done in two weeks or less. Unfortunately, this pattern sets you up for burnout. If you are dealing with PMS during one two-week stretch of the month (which takes a lot of energy) and overworking at the office the other two weeks, you are depriving yourself of any good time at all. During your symptom-free phase, see if you are taking extra work home on a regular basis. Are you skipping your breaks and working extra long hours? If you find this to be the case, take steps to break that pattern. Otherwise, you place yourself in a no-win situation.

$Q.$ **I have called my husband home from work at times because I simply couldn't cope. Do other husbands miss much work because of their wives' PMS?**

$A.$ There are plenty of men who have missed work because of their wives' PMS. The situation you describe illustrates the far-reaching effects of PMS on families and the workplace. If more husbands or significant others were to address the issue of PMS, there would be far more interest in encouraging further research.

Q. Why isn't PMS a subject taught or brought up in sex education classes in high schools?

A. I think the fact that PMS isn't taught in class is just another reflection of the lack of awareness by the general public. Once everyone is better informed about this serious problem, I think we will see PMS included in most health curricula.

Q. If this had been a "man's issue," don't you agree that research, funding and relief would have come about long ago?

A. While there is little doubt that PMS sufferers have been called "typically female," I think both men and women have been operating under the assumption that women are changeable and irritable by nature. Even though some people may see PMS as a "woman's issue," I would have to say that it has such far-reaching effects on a woman's family that everyone would benefit from viewing it as a "family issue."

Q. Am I a traitor if I acknowledge PMS?

A. Obviously, I don't think so, or I would consider myself a traitor, but it is very important that we address the political question of PMS. A surprising number of women feel we are doing ourselves a disservice to even acknowledge PMS as a real and sometimes crippling reality. They think this supports the argument that women should never hold positions of power because of their "raging hormones." I strongly disagree with this argument. We would not have any trouble with a male, diabetic president so long as he was on insulin therapy, controlling his diet and exercising. The situation is analogous to a woman who has PMS. She has the ability to hold a position of power provided she controls her PMS with diet, exercise, vitamins and medical intervention if indicated. PMS is not an untreatable condition. It does not render a woman helpless and incapable. Therefore, I would have to say that by not acknowledging that PMS exists, women will be deprived of the help they need to improve their careers and relationships. I use myself as an example. I know that I would never have achieved positive relationships at home or success in my profession had I pretended that PMS didn't exist. By identifying the syndrome in myself and getting effective treatment for it, I have achieved many goals that seemed absolutely impossible before.

Q. Are my legal rights diminished because I have PMS?

A. Probably not. My legal adviser confirms that PMS has not been used as a legal defense in the United States nor has it been used against any individual. To our knowledge, this has not yet been tested in the courts.

Q. Is there any organization to contact if I feel I am being discriminated against in the workplace because of PMS?

A. That's a good question; any form of discrimination needs to be addressed. If you feel you you have been the victim of discrimination, I suggest you contact a lawyer. At this particular time, I know of no organization that specifically represents the rights of PMS sufferers.

Q. **I find it somewhat difficult to admit to people that I have a tendency toward PMS. I had to fill out a new insurance form and felt morally obligated to mention it. I felt embarrassed when the male insurance agent read my statement in front of my male boss.**

A. Embarrassment about PMS is not unusual. I believe that it will become less embarrassing to talk about your own PMS when society as a whole accepts it more readily. The actions of your insurance agent were unacceptable and demonstrated an insensitivity and lack of professionalism. Every person dealing with a medical problem of any type has the right to privacy. In addressing the subject of PMS, we also need to be aware of the skepticism with which it is viewed by many of the people with whom we live and work.

Q. **Should I educate myself about PMS or am I merely talking myself into thinking that I have it as some doctors suggest?**

A. I believe that education is paramount. I don't think that by educating yourself you are in any way trying to convince yourself that you have PMS. It is important to read objective information and to document daily what your symptoms are so that you can get as clear a picture as possible of your condition. I would avoid any doctor who suggests that by educating yourself about PMS you are only trying to convince yourself that you have it.

Q. Do you think the public will become more aware of this medical problem that affects so many women?

A. Yes. I see the PMS movement as a grass roots movement. It is very similar to the situation that existed when Lamaze was first introduced in this country. When women became educated about the process of giving birth and were encouraged to actively participate, they began to realize that they benefited greatly. I believe that as women with PMS become aware that this syndrome is not necessarily "part of being a woman," they will respond by telling family members, doctors and other women, and they will insist on effective help.

Q. Have any well known women publicly discussed their PMS?

A. I don't know of any celebrities who have come forward and revealed their own stories regarding PMS. However, the book and movie *Mommy Dearest* certainly suggests that the actress Joan Crawford may have had PMS.

Q. Is PMS widely recognized by doctors?

A. Recognition is increasing, but we have a long way to go in this area.

Q. I recently had a very damaging experience with a psychiatrist who claimed to understand PMS but in reality did not. Are counselors (psychiatrists and psychologists) being trained to understand what PMS is and what it is not?

A. Some medical and graduate schools do a better job of teaching about PMS than others. As a general rule, the training of mental health professionals does not include much information on PMS. Most of the professionals who deal with PMS have learned about it from seminars, keeping up with new research findings and their own experience with patients.

Q. **What can I do to aid in educating the general public and the medical community concerning PMS?**

A. This is a most difficult question because it involves your personal exposure if you believe you have PMS. First, you may need to conquer the feeling that PMS women are inferior in any way. Make statements that portray PMS as a controllable syndrome. Then take every opportunity available to convey to the general public your success in gaining control of the syndrome. The best way to impact the medical community is by informing your doctor that you will seek out a physician who takes your complaints and self-observations seriously.

Q. **How much research is being done on PMS?**

A. There are many kinds of research currently being conducted in the medical, psychological and psychosocial areas of PMS. Please consult the appendix of this book for further information on this subject.

Q. Are there any beneficial aspects of PMS?

A. Dr. Michelle Harrison has done a great deal of research in this area and has found that some women's creativity and abilities and physical strength are actually heightened during PMS days. You might want to read her work, *SELF-HELP FOR PREMENSTRUAL SYNDROME*, Matrix Press, 1984 for further information.

PART III

GETTING SOME HELP

Eight

WHAT CAN I DO TO HELP MYSELF?

Q. Can PMS symptoms be cured?

A. I would hesitate to use the word "cure" in relation to PMS. I would say that it is perfectly reasonable for a woman who has PMS to expect the symptoms to be significantly alleviated so that she can be in control of her PMS, rather than her PMS being in control of her.

Q. How do I get motivated to work on controlling the symptoms?

A. It's easier for you to get motivated during the symptom-free time of your cycle. Do a "reality check" and tell yourself that you would like to feel this great all month long. By knowing that self-help measures will make the good times last longer, you will set the stage for the best possible chance for success. Finally, seek the help of a support system whether that means friends, family, mutual support group or physician to help you if you run into problems along the way.

Q. Are vitamins really that important?

A. Absolutely! Your diet has a significant effect on how you feel. A woman with a hormonal imbalance needs extra vitamin requirements to maintain a nutritional equilibrium.

Q. What vitamins should I be taking if I have PMS?

A. There are two commercial products on the market which I think are excellent. One is called Procycle and one is Optivite. They are both vitamin, mineral and trace element supplement formulated for women with PMS.

Q. Is it true that B-complex vitamins are connected to hormonal levels?

A. Yes they are. B-complex vitamins are important in regulating estrogen levels. Estrogen becomes elevated when you are deficient in the B-complex vitamins. Because PMS is caused by high levels of estrogen and low levels of progesterone, a B-complex deficiency could lead to an exacerbation of PMS symptoms.

Q. Please explain the diverse thinking on vitamins and PMS. I was told by one OB/GYN to take 500 mg. of vitamin B6 twice a day and

have been doing so for a year. Recently, another doctor told me nobody should take B6 because of complications in the nervous system. Who is right?

A. I don't agree with either doctor. Vitamin B6 is a natural diuretic that helps release the excess fluid buildup in your body that may occur during the premenstrual phase. Vitamin B6 does not work well unless it is used with the other B vitamins. That's why I suggest a B-complex if you want to increase your dosage of B6. Even though B6 is a water soluble vitamin, too much of it can affect the nervous system adversely. I think that 500 mg. twice a day is too much B6; I suggest a single dosage of 200 to 300 mg. of B6 per day.

Q. **Why would I need to get rid of excess water in my body if I have PMS?**

A. Most people want to get rid of the excess fluid because it makes them feel uncomfortable. Bloated abdomens and sore breasts are the most common manifestations of fluid retention. While these symptoms are not life-threatening, they can be unpleasant.

Q. **Why don't doctors advocate the use of B-complex vitamins for water retention instead of prescribing "water pills?"**

A. I agree with you that a B-complex vitamin would be a more reasonable suggestion than a prescription diuretic. Physicians may be unaware that B-complex vitamins work in this way. I would also suggest pink, unsweetened grapefruit juice or lemon juice and water as good, natural diuretics.

Q. My friend was told to take large doses of magnesium in order to alleviate her PMS symptoms. How does magnesium help?

A. Magnesium deficiencies can lead to fluid retention, cyclic constipation and nervous tension. Therefore, it is important to make sure you are getting adequate amounts of this mineral. The correct calcium/magnesium balance must be maintained. One without the other is going to sabotage your efforts. The correct ratio is twice as much calcium as magnesium. Magnesium can also be obtained from your diet. Foods rich in magnesium are green vegetables, nuts, seeds, whole grains, beans, peas and lentils.

Q. What role does zinc play in the PMS picture?

A. Your body needs zinc to resist infection. In view of the fact that many women with PMS complain of increased incidence of catching contagious diseases, such as colds and flu, during their premenstrual phase, it is important to make sure you are getting adequate zinc.

Q. I've heard that women with PMS are told to eat six meals a day. I would weigh 200 pounds if I did that! What do you suggest as a reasonable diet for PMS?

A. Eating six meals a day is an excellent idea for a woman trying to control PMS. That does not mean that she is eating six full meals. It does mean, however, that she will control her blood sugar level by eating frequently and eating healthful foods. The following is an example of a daily PMS diet:

Breakfast:	Whole grain cereal with low fat milk (2% butterfat)
	A medium banana
	Herbal tea
Snack:	One pear
	Two to three low-salt Triscuits or brown rice crackers
Lunch:	Tuna salad sandwich on whole wheat bread
	Sliced tomato
	Salt-free sparkling water or pink unsweetened grapefruit juice
Dinner:	Baked chicken
	Squash
	Whole wheat roll
	Tossed salad with low-fat, low-salt dressing
Snack:	Unsalted, unbuttered popcorn

Reduce your intake of caffeine, alcohol, salt, sugar and sodas (especially colas and artificial sweeteners). Increase your intake of fresh fruits, vegetables and complex carbohydrates (whole grains). Dietary measures are most effective when carried out all month long. You are less likely to be motivated to make dietary changes during your premenstrual phase. Therefore, by sticking to your diet during the symptom-free time of the cycle, you will enhance the chances that you will continue through your PMS phase.

Q. **I take a PMS vitamin which I buy over-the-counter. A flyer packed into the bottle outlines a diet based on the research of Dr. Guy Abraham. The diet recommends a high fiber low-fat regimen. It also leans heavily on the consumption of whole grains (like barley and millet) and dried peas and beans for vegetable protein. What are the advantages of such a diet?**

A. The vitamin you are describing is Optivites developed by Dr. Guy Abraham. The diet he suggests will benefit you because it concentrates on the consumption of complex carbohydrates which are rich energy sources for women with PMS. Complex carbohydrates sustain the blood sugar level over long periods of time. Dr. Abraham's dietary suggestions are excellent.

Q. **Today's foods are full of additives, preservative, food colorings and the like. How do I eat to improve my PMS?**

A. You bring up some good points which show why eating to alleviate PMS symptoms can take more energy than you think. However, it is well worth the effort. Become a label reader to determine which foods are appropriate for you. Ingredients are listed on product labels from the highest percentage to the lowest percentage. Therefore, if salt, sugar or other additives are near the top of the list, I would avoid the product. Use as many fresh fruits and vegetables as possible. By eating fresh produce you cut down on any additives while you satisfy your hunger.

Q. Which snacks are good for me?

A. Try combining half a cup of salted sunflower seeds with an equal quantity of unsalted seeds. The same holds true for other nuts. This combination can satisfy your need for something crunchy with only half the salt.

Fresh fruits and vegetables are always a good idea. Half a banana, a few strips of green pepper or an apple are excellent ideas. Be sure to add one or two low-salt whole grain crackers to stablize the blood sugar level while you are satisfying your taste for something sweet.

Remember that you don't have to eat a lot, but you do have to eat frequently to help stabilize the blood sugar level. Of course if healthy snacks aren't around, you can usually be tempted by unhealthful ones. For example, if you don't make a habit of having low-salt, whole grain crackers at work, the candy and chips in the vending machine are going to look very appealing. Do yourself a favor and bring a week's supply of snacks on the first day of the work week.

Q. I can't stay away from chocolate. Are there any healthful substitutes?

A. Chocolate can be a problem because it contains sugar, caffeine and fat. Unfortunately, I don't know of any substitute. Small, frequent meals during the day can help control your craving. I am also a firm believer in eating fruit when you desire something sweet. As a professional who deals with PMS women and as a past PMS woman myself, I would rather see a woman eating grapes (which are very sweet with the natural sugar fructose) than a candy bar. When I was craving something sweet, such as chocolate, I would have driven a hundred miles to buy a Snickers bar if I didn't have access to fresh fruit. Interestingly, chocolate contains magnesium. It is possible that you are craving this sweet to satisfy a magnesium deficiency. Make sure that you are getting adequate magnesium in your diet through the proper nutritional supplements.

Q. Why should I avoid caffeine?

A. A woman with PMS needs to stabilize her blood sugar level because fluctuations can result in feelings of irritability, headaches and food cravings. She should avoid substances that can cause her blood sugar level to skyrocket and then plummet. Caffeine affects blood sugar levels dramatically. Caffeine is also directly correlated to breast soreness.

In addition, caffeine is a stimulant. If you already feel tense, you don't need the additional stimulant effect of caffeine.

Q. When my ex-boyfriend and I started living together, we'd begin every morning with a pot, sometimes two, of thick, black coffee. During this time, I began to behave erratically. My doctor suggested I remove caffeine from my diet. I have also ended the relationship with my boyfriend, and for the past six months, I've been relatively sypmtom-free.

A. It sounds as if caffeine coupled with a difficult relationship were real problems for you. Two pots of strong coffee in the morning will create tidal waves for a PMS woman because of the fluctuation in her blood sugar. You have been very successful with the self-help measures. You eliminated two irritants from your life: caffeine and the relationship.

Q. **I'm trying to give up coffee, but I'm having a hard time. Do you have any suggestions?**

A. There are two approaches to giving up caffeine. The first is to cut down slowly by combining equal parts of caffeinated and decaffeinated coffee for a week. The following week, you can reduce the caffeinated coffee to only a quarter of the brew. By the third week, you should be off caffeine completely. If you are a moderate to heavy user of caffeine, this approach may work well for you. Of course, you may also choose to go cold turkey and give up caffeine all at once. Remember to substitute rather than eliminate completely. Replace your source of caffeine with decaffeinated coffee or herbal teas.

Q. **I only drink two to three cups of coffee a day. When I tried to eliminate caffeine, I got such terrible headaches that I had to go back to it. What can I take for those headaches? Over-the-counter drugs don't work.**

A. You are having caffeine withdrawal headaches. As you have noticed, over-the-counter remedies do little to alleviate this discomfort. When you get a caffeine withdrawal headache, take one or two swallows of caffeinated coffee to relieve the pain. Over the course of ten to fourteen days, your body should be weaned from caffeine and the headaches will no longer be a problem. Caffeine withdrawal headaches are a painful warning of the physical and psychological dependency we can develop with caffeine.

A word of caution here: you may also experience some dullness and lack of energy when you eliminate caffeine from your diet. You were getting energy from the caffeine and it is important to replace that energy source with another healthier one. Try eating a piece of fresh fruit and a small amount of a complex carbohydrate (like whole grain crackers) to give you that energy you used to get from caffeine.

Q. **I know there is caffeine in coffee. I've heard it is hidden in other foods. What else should I watch out for?**

A. Caffeine is most commonly found in:
- Tea
- Coffee
- Soft drinks
- Chocolate

Q. **Why do I gain five to ten pounds, usually in puffiness, before my period starts? I go back to my normal weight once it starts.**

A. Many women report premenstrual weight fluctuations. The "puffiness" that you notice may be due to increased fluid retention. Salt causes the body to retain excess fluid. Curtail the amount of salt you eat. In fact, it's not a bad idea to limit salt all month long since you may not be motivated to make dietary changes during your premenstrual phase. By decreasing your salt intake during the non-premenstrual phase of your cycle, you are more likely to continue this pattern into your premenstrual phase.

$Q.$ **Sometimes during the warm weather, I get cravings for salt. Is it possible to be completely depleted of salt?**

$A.$ Given the American diet, it is not likely that you will be completely depleted of salt. That is not to say that it is impossible. Even if you eliminate cooking with salt or add it to foods, it is still present in many foods. In fact, it is fairly difficult to avoid salt entirely. However, in the warm weather you are constantly losing body fluids through perspiration. Increase your intake of fluids if you notice this happening rather than increasing your salt consumption.

$Q.$ **Besides cutting down on salt, how can I get rid of premenstrual bloating?**

$A.$ You can use the natural diurectics that I suggested earlier in the chapter. Also look for "hidden salt" in packaged foods that you eat regularly whose salt content you may not even consider. A good example of this is cheese.

Some other examples of high salt foods are:
• Salted crackers and chips
• Canned vegetables that don't say "low sodium"

- Frozen foods such as TV dinners and frozen pizza
- Butter
- Cottage cheese
- Salsa

Replace high salt foods with these:
- Unsalted or lightly salted crackers
- Canned vegetables that are labeled "low sodium"
- Light and unsalted butter or margarine

Remember, every food label containing the word sodium, such as monosodium glutamate or bisodium carbonate, is high in sodium and should be avoided.

Q. How do I eliminate salt from the food I cook?

A. Spices are a great way to flavor food while you cut down on the use of salt. There are so many herbs and seasonings that it would be impossible to list them all. Visit your local grocery store and browse the aisle that has all of the spices. With the awareness of the dangers of salt, many combination spices are available which blend ingredients such as onion, garlic, parsley, basil, celery, lemon peel, cayenne pepper, paprika, oregano and thyme. These really add zest to your cooking without aggravating your PMS symptoms.

Q. My appetite is out of control. Why and what can I do?

A. Many women with PMS experience fluctuating blood sugar levels that throw appetite out of control. The best way to deal with a fluctuating blood sugar level is to work toward stabilizing it. Eliminate foods which cause big dips such as sugar, caffeine and alcohol. Eat small meals frequently thoughout the day, concentrating on healthful foods. Try a fruit snack combined with a small amount of complex carbohydrate.

Q. I have PMS and I also have low blood sugar. Are PMS symptoms and the symptoms associated with low blood sugar similar?

A. Some of the symptoms of low blood sugar and PMS coincide. Irritiability, fatigue, loss of concentration and headaches occur in both situations. During the premenstrual phase of the cycle, your diet concerns are a top priority.

Q. I get shaky and hungry just before my period and crave chocolate a good week before it starts. This always sabotages my activities to keep my weight down. What can I do to end the food cravings?

A. Eat frequently, throughout the day. The general rule of thumb is: Don't go longer than three hours without food. By eating healthful foods frequently you help keep your blood sugar level stable and minimize your food cravings. You also increase your mental alertness. Substitute a piece of fresh fruit for a cookie when you get a craving for something sweet.

Q. How often is treating yourself to some forbidden food too often?

A. I guess that depends on your definition of "forbidden" and "often." Although I'm not a purist in the diet category, I realize that I have a high price to pay for eating sweets. In view of the consequences, I wouldn't call it a real treat. It is easier to stick to my diet (limiting my sugar and salt) if I do it on a regular basis. Why not think of a treat as something good for you, like a crab salad? Then you can treat yourself as often as you like.

Q. Why does going on an eating binge do such terrible things to me?

A. The psychological aspect of bingeing complicates the picture. Dietary considerations aside, when you binge, you can become depressed because you think of yourself as losing control. PMS also involves loss of control. All of this is compounded by remorse, failure and guilt.

Q. Why do I have such difficulty controlling my weight?

A. This is a knotty problem. There are physiological and psychological issues to consider.

Blood sugar levels fluctuate tremendously during the premenstrual phase of the cycle. This can lead to cravings for foods such as sugar and refined carbohydrates. Obviously, if your appetite increases and you respond with junk food, you will tend to put on a few extra pounds.

Premenstrual bloating is another major cause for weight fluctuation. Your body may retain extra fluid premenstrually, which can result in extra pounds. Therefore, it is very important to avoid salt all month long, but especially during the premenstrual phase.

When you give in to a food craving, you become depressed. An attitude of "I've blown my diet already, why should I try anymore?" is very defeating and needs to be recognized as a common trap for PMS women. One binge leads to another, causing you to feel defeated.

Q. **When I have PMS, I get so depressed all I want to do is eat to make myself feel better. When I overeat, I sink further. How do I get out of this trap?**

A. Overeating causes physical discomfort and can certainly be depressing. Make sure that you don't have junk food available in your home so you won't be tempted. Keep healthful foods available so that when your appetite increases you are more likely to reach for fruit than candy. If you do find yourself bingeing on a sugary treat, it is not the time to heap guilt on yourself; you are going to feel bad enough from the blood sugar level drop. Think of ways other than food to make yourself feel better and keep a list of alternatives like calling a friend or going for a walk. Whatever you do, don't sit around and think about food.

Q. **I have a very bad attitude about my body image. I don't think I'm overweight, but I still hate the way I look when I have my period or PMS.**

A. You are not alone! Many women are unhappy with the way they perceive their body image during the premenstrual phase. This may come from the water weight gain which is so common during this time. Bloating of the abdomen may cause you to feel like you are in the first trimester of pregnancy! How can you feel better? You may want to withdraw during the premenstrual phase. If public excercising feels unacceptable, try excercising in the privacy of your own home. Some floor excercises or even running in place will probably give you more energy and lighten your spirits. Your attitude about body image will improve after a vigorous workout. At least it's a step in the right direction.

Q. **Why is exercise important?**

A. Exercise is very important in the overall self-help program for a PMS woman. It not only gives you a physical workout, but allows you to release emotions through physical activity rather than angry outbursts.

Q. **How does exercise help in treating PMS symptoms?**

A. It makes a tremendous difference! Overall, good health will help minimize any physical problem. If your body is in good condition from a regular exercise program, even lower back pain will be less problematic. Exercise is an ideal way to rid the body of the heightened stress that occurs during those PMS days. However, it does need to be considered on an individual basis. A woman with

PMS should exercise at least three times a week for no less than one half hour each time.

Q. How does exercise make me feel better? I'd rather be a couch potato.

A. Exercise causes the brain to secrete endorphins, which are amino acids with analgesic properties that relieve pain and elevate your mood. This alone can produce a feeling of well-being. On the other hand, lack of exercise depresses the body. Proper, regular exercise energizes and relaxes you.

Q. Do you recommend any specific kind of exercise? Is swimming better than yoga?

A. I would answer with a qualified yes. I do recommend an aerobic exercise, one which elevates your heartbeat like jogging, brisk walking or tennis. However, some women prefer the stretching, centering effects of yoga. I certainly would recommend any form of exercise over none at all.

Q. I hate to exercise! How do I get going?

A. Start your exercise program during the symptom-free time of your cycle. You are more likely to be successful during your premenstrual phase if a routine is established at this high motivation time. Second, choose a form of exercise that you enjoy. If you never liked to swim, this is not the time to start swimming. Exercise does not have to be painful! A brisk walk in the fresh air for thirty minutes can cause an elevated pulse rate that can be very effective and invigorating. Third, ask someone to help motivate you when you are feeling sluggish and down. A friend or family member could accompany you or just encourage you to take a ten minute walk (which may end up being thirty minutes because it feels so good once you get started). Remember, the hardest part of exercise is getting started!

Nine

MEDICAL ALTERNATIVES FOR PMS

Q. **How do I know if my PMS is serious enough to warrant medical treatment?**

A. If PMS is significant enough to be affecting your personal and work life, I suggest that the first line of treatment be self-help, which includes diet, exercise and vitamins. If those measures do not significantly alleviate your symptoms after two months, consider further medical treatment. Be very careful in choosing the health care practitioner you'll be working with. Make sure that his or her beliefs correspond with yours. Remember that a team approach is essential. You are a vital part of that team (see Chapter Ten).

Q. **What are PMS treatments?**

A. Treatments for PMS range widely. Some doctors still prescribe tranquilizers, birth control pills or hysterectomies while others recommend natural progesterone replacement therapy. I believe that diet, exercise and vitamin therapy is the best first line of treatment. If this approach does not significantly alleviate the symptoms, then natural progesterone replacement therapy ought to be considered.

Q. What is the quickest cure for PMS?

A. There are no quick cures for PMS. The best treatment is charting your symptoms and self-help measures practiced over a period of time. If satisfactory results are not achieved, medical intervention should be used to augment the self-help measures. When you appreciate how long you have had to deal with PMS, treatment time will seem short in comparison.

Q. Without treatment to alleviate PMS symptoms, do you think a woman would feel better eventually?

A. I believe that if a woman has significant PMS and is not doing anything to better the situation, she is on a disaster course. If she can make it to and through menopause, her hormonal imbalance will eventually even out, and the symptoms of PMS may subside. However, it can be a long and rocky road, and I certainly would suggest that every PMS woman actively try to help herself instead of waiting it out.

Q. After documenting her PMS symptoms and beginning treatment for them, my sister

started to deny she ever had it. After a while she discontinued treatment. Why would this happen?

A. Some women are still working through the denial that can be a part of PMS. However, if they discontinue treatment, their symptoms usually return, and they are confronted with the reality of the situation. Most will then return to the treatment plan. It may take your sister several setbacks before she finally accepts the fact that she feels better when she takes care of herself. One of my patients once said, "I went through doing it right and doing it wrong, and I saw the difference, but I still tested it."

Q. **Is there any medicine that can make PMS easier to deal with?**

A. If self-help measures do not significantly alleviate the problem of PMS, natural progesterone replacement therapy has proven to be helpful for many women.

Q. **You have advocated natural progesterone. Is there an artificial progesterone. If so, why is the natural substance better for me to use?**

A. Natural progesterone is called progesterone. The synthetic is called progestogen. Progestogen diminishes the natual progesterone that your body produces. Since PMS is thought to be caused by insufficient progesterone, anything that reduces an already low level is likely to make the situation worse. This seems to occur with many PMS patients. If you are interested in using progesterone for the treatment of PMS, avoid the synthetic form.

Q. How is progesterone administered?

A. Natural progesterone is most often administered in the form of a suppository (rectal or vaginal) or a liquid that is inserted rectally. Shots are available, but they are expensive and painful.

Q. Why are progesterone suppositories more effective than other ways of taking this drug?

A. The vaginal and rectal mucous membrane are very rich in blood supply. By using a vaginal or rectal suppository, the medication is rapidly absorbed and enters your bloodstream effectively.

Q. When is the best time of day to take the progesterone suppositories?

A. You should take progesterone during your waking hours. Start out the day with your first dosage and take subsequent doses throughout the day. Taking progesterone only before going to bed doesn't bring about the desired results.

Q. Why doesn't the FDA approve progesterone? Is it a safe drug?

A. While progesterone is an FDA approved drug and is available in the United States, the FDA has not approved it as a treatment for PMS. For instance, Motrin is an anti-prostaglandin that is frequently prescribed for menstrual cramps. Initially, it was formulated for the treatment of arthritis and was approved by the FDA for that purpose. When women used this drug for arthritis, it was discovered that the anti-prostaglandin relieved menstrual cramps as well. Motrin is now being prescribed for cramps. Progesterone occurs in very high levels during normal pregnancy without causing any negative side effects. When you take progesterone for PMS, you are not introducing any foreign substance into your body. Even though all medications should be taken cautiously, one of the advantages of progesterone is its lack of significant side effects.

Q. How long does a woman have to take progesterone before she finds relief?

A. You will experience results from the natural progesterone during the first month of therapy. However, I should caution that progesterone is not a quick solution. Your health care practitioner may need to adjust the days and dosages of the progesterone before optimum results can be achieved. Remember, all self-help measures should be used to optimize the effects of progesterone therapy.

Q. Can I become addicted to progesterone?

A. Progesterone is not an addictive substance.

Q. Can you overdose on progesterone?

A. Dr. Katharina Dalton, England's foremost PMS expert, says that a woman who has experienced a pregnancy cannot overdose on progesterone since her body has already experienced high levels of it during pregnancy. A woman who has never experienced a pregnancy can overdose on progesterone but not in a life-threatening way. If she does take too much, she may experience some restlessness and a high energy level which is sometimes referred to as euphoria.

Q. There is a great deal of concern among doctors regarding progesterone. Can you explain why it is so hard to get?

A. Progesterone is available in pharmacies across the country. Many doctors are unfamiliar with progesterone, and therefore, are reluctant to work with it. If the physician is unfamiliar with progesterone and is unwilling to learn about its proper administration, he or she should not prescribe it.

Q. I think I'm approaching the menopausal stage. Am I too old to benefit from progesterone therapy?

A. Not at all! If you and your health care practitioner agree that self-help measures are not adequately alleviating your symptoms, progesterone therapy is an approach to consider.

Q. I'm on progesterone, and it isn't working. Why not?

$A.$ You don't mention whether you are using progesterone as a part of a total program combined with self-help measures or not. If not, your diet may be sabotaging you. However, if you are using the correct self-help in conjunction with your therapy, you need to be evaluated by a health care practitioner who is familiar with progesterone therapy. If your progesterone is not taken at the right time of day, in the correct dosage and starting at the appropriate time of your cycle, it is be destined to fail. While I don't see progesterone as a cure-all for all PMS women, it will alleviate PMS symptoms in many sufferers when it is used correctly.

$Q.$ **Why isn't there more pharmacological help available for PMS patients?**

$A.$ There is good pharmacological help available. One excellent resource is Madison Pharmacy Associates. They publish a newsletter every two months and give excellent referrals. Registered pharmacists are available to answer your questions at 1 800-558-7046.

$Q.$ **Are other countries more advanced in dealing with PMS? Do they have effective medications that might not yet be approved in the U.S.?**

$A.$ I am not aware of any new medication that is being used in other countries.

$Q.$ **Four years ago I saw a doctor to whom I was referred for my PMS. He put me on a** medication that I took for almost a year until I read in a book that it was a mood elevator for people with mental problems. Since I am not (and never have been) mentally disabled, I quit taking it immediately. Isn't there some natural way I can get treatment for this problem?

A. It is unfortunate that you dealt with a doctor who gave you a mood elevator for PMS. That type of drug will not take care of your problem as you have already discovered. Even though it may have been implied that PMS is a mental problem, this is not the case. Follow my suggestions in Chapter Ten to seek out another doctor.

Q. Do you feel that tranquilizers are ever warranted in the treatment of PMS?

A. I believe strongly that the use of tranquilizers to treat PMS on a regular basis is counterproductive. The potential of abusing such drugs is very high. If a physician suggests the regular use of a tranquilizer, he or she is promoting the idea that PMS is all in a woman's mind. On the other hand, if a woman is in crisis and is threatening suicide, I do not oppose the use of tranquilizers on a short-term emergency basis.

Q. I take a low-dose tranquilizer two to three days a month to help control my PMS. I have altered my diet, and I excercise regularly. I must say these measures have helped a great deal. However, for those two to three days I am only able to manage things with the tranquilizer. How do I guard against addiction?

Sometimes during overly stressful months, the two to three days turns into six to ten days.

A. You are playing with fire. Most tranquilizers are addictive. The only way to guard against addiction is to discontinue using the tranquilizer on such a regular basis and look for some other solution for your PMS. I certainly commend you for your efforts in altering your diet and excercising regularly. Why not add a vitamin supplement? Explore other medical interventions rather than tranquilizers if the self-help measures are not adequately alleviating your PMS symptoms.

Q. **I've heard of some herbs such as Dong Quai that are helpful for hormonal problems. What do you think?**

A. Herbs are a form of medication. Many of our over-the-counter and prescription pharmaceutical products are derived from herbs, as well as other sources.

A word of caution here: you may assume that since a herb is a "natural" substance, we can't use too much of it, and it can't harm us in any way. That can be a problem. Herbs are medications that should be treated with the same caution as any other drug. Too much is unknown about herbs for me to comfortably condone their general use as a treatment.

Q. **Is it true that marijuana is an effective treatment for PMS?**

A. No, it is not true. Many of my patients who

have used marijuana say that it makes them very nervous and paranoid.

Q. A friend of mine takes oil of evening primrose for her PMS. Is it effective?

A. Oil of evening primrose is also called efamol, a substance high in vitamin E. From my clinical experience, it seems that women who take efamol don't enjoy dramatic relief from their PMS symptoms. In theory, it is speculated that efamol could be effective. It has a sort of a domino effect. Efamol may increase prostaglandin production. This, in turn, could decrease the prolactin level. Lower levels of prolactin are thought to increase the progesterone level.

Q. My baby was born two years ago, and I'm still secreting milk, although I am no longer nursing. Is there any connection between this condition and my PMS? Is there any drug I can take to correct the problem?

A. Since you are still secreting milk, it is possible that your prolactin level is elevated. You may want to check with your physician to have the prolactin checked. High prolactin can create problems in the PMS woman by lowering the progesterone level. Your first line of attack is to treat the prolactin. For this problem, most physicians prescribe the drug bromocriptine sold as Parlodel in the pharmacy.

Q. I've seen some over-the-counter preparations for PMS. Do you recommend them?

A. No, I don't. These products usually contain an analgesic (pain killer), a very mild diuretic and an antihistamine (to make you drowsy). I would much rather see a woman using diet, excercise and vitamins to treat her PMS than preparations such as these.

Q. Should I have a hysterectomy?

A. Hysterectomies do not cure PMS. The term hysterectomy refers to a procedure in which the uterus is removed, but the ovaries are left intact. Research shows that in some cases, but not all, the ovaries continue to function following a hysterectomy. If the ovaries function, the same hormonal imbalances can be experienced after the hysterectomy as before. If the ovaries don't function, a hormonal imbalance will also ensue. In either case, a hysterectomy for PMS can create more problems than it solves.

Q. My doctor says he can't find anything wrong with me physically. He says that PMS can be controlled by having an operation to stop my periods. Is he right?

A. No. The operation your doctor is referring to is called a hysterectomy. It involves the removal of the uterus so, obviously, no menstrual flow would be experienced. Even though we call PMS premenstrual syndrome, the syndrome can also take place in the absence of menstruation. Hysterectomies have been reported to exacerbate PMS symptoms in some women. Measures such as diet, exercise, vitamin therapy and other medical

135

treatment to control PMS are most successful in controlling PMS. You need to try options that improve your situation, not make it worse.

Q. **After twenty years of seeking help I was finally diagnosed at age forty-three as having severe PMS. I had a hysterectomy at age forty-one and since my ovaries were not removed, I still have PMS. My problem is that I have no way of knowing where I am in my cycle in order to be on guard after ovulation. By the time I'm aware that it's premenstrual time, it's too late. The only possible solution I've been able to come up with is to be on a PMS diet constantly. Charting has helped a little bit, but it isn't entirely reliable since my cycle used to be anywhere from twenty-eight to thirty-three days. How can women who have undergone a hysterectomy determine their PMS days?**

A. Try a basal temperature chart to determine ovulation. When your basal temperature rises and stays high, you can be reasonably sure that ovulation has occured. After charting this for a few months, you will discover that you ovulate about the same time each month. This information will help you in determining when your premenstrual phase begins. There's no harm in staying on your PMS diet all month long to further assist controlling your symptoms.

Q. **Why wouldn't removal of the ovaries and the uterus cure PMS?**

A. The type of surgery you are describing is a very dramatic step to take in trying to control PMS. Indeed, you would be trading one imbalance for another. The removal of these vital organs will throw you into a "surgical menopause." You will require hormonal replacement therapy to restore the body's hormonal balance. You cannot cure PMS by removing either the uterus or the ovaries.

Ten

CREATING A SUPPORT SYSTEM

Q. **Where can I find help?**

A. Look to your personal and professional support systems, and let those people know you need assistance. If self-help isn't effective, ask your health care practitioner about medical options. Bring your charts with you to clarify the severity and timing of your symptoms. Be sure to educate yourself so that you know what to ask for.

Q. **Can my family doctor be my PMS doctor?**

A. I would have to answer with a qualified yes. If your physician seems knowledgeable and demonstrates a genuine concern for the problem, listen carefully. At the same time, do some of your own research by reading the published information on PMS and talking to other individuals who have the syndrome. Be willing to express your own ideas on

PMS to your health care practitioner. The end result should be an effective team effort. If you are dissatisfied with your doctor's approach, you have the option of seeking a second or third opinion. Trust yourself and your instincts. If the doctor you see first doesn't feel right, don't be afraid to look elsewhere.

Q. I'm moving out of state. How will I find a doctor who believes that PMS exists and is willing to treat it?

A. Word of mouth recommendations tend to be the best. If you don't think that you are getting reliable information, you might consider calling the PMS Clinic in Boulder, Colorado at (303) 440-7100 for a listing of health care practitioners in your area whom you can query regarding their PMS policy. The doctor you choose should be open and willing to discuss his or her approach towards PMS with you. If not, continue looking.

Q. My doctor maintains that PMS is a catchall and that there is no such thing. I know from watching my own cycle that I have emotional changes no matter what he says. What should I do to get help with my PMS? I have already altered my diet. I am exercising and taking vitamins.

A. Unfortunately, there are still doctors who think PMS is a catchall term. It is important to trust yourself. If you have been charting yourself and have observed a pattern, you probabley do have

PMS. I encourage you to continue with your self-help measures. You may wish to find another doctor. There is nothing more important than creating a professional support system which truly supports you!

Q. How can I seek out a therapist who understands PMS?

A. After your initial meeting with a therapist, you should get a feel for his or her attitude as it relates to your condition. If you sense that there is a genuine understanding, great! If understanding and knowledge are not present, don't be afraid to look for another therapist. Your instincts are often reliable in situations like these.

Q. How is PMS treated by counselors?

A. I don't think it is fair to make general statements about all counselors. Some counselors still treat PMS as it has been treated historically. They ignore it, or they call it "part of being a woman." Other, better informed counselors pay attention to the fact that their clients' behavior seems to follow a regular pattern. They include the problem of PMS in the total treatment plan.

Q. I have PMS but live in a state that has no clinics or doctors who seem to know about PMS. Where do I go for help?

A. The library is the first stop. Educate yourself about PMS and furnish information (medical journal articles) to your physician. Then you stand a better chance of enlisting your doctor's cooperation. If you can't find the information you are looking for, call or write the PMS Clinic, Boulder, Colorado. The number is (303) 440-7100.

Q. **I found your book *PMS: A Positive Program To Gain Control* in the library recently and was so glad to discover that what I've been feeling is a real medical problem and not a mental one. It helps to know that I am not alone. I've been to two doctors who told me I was imagining my symptoms. I'm skeptical of doctors, but I need help badly to save my family life.**

I am 31, married and have three girls. I had a tubal ligation three years ago. After seeing PMS discussed on TV, I made a chart for four months. I have all the symptoms, some very severely. I feel good seven to ten days after the third day of my period. People make me feel very bad about myself because I'm not supposed to be this way just because it is "my time of the month."

A. Many women find themselves in the same dilemma as you. The PMS Clinic and I will do our best to put you in touch with someone in your area who can effectively work with you.

Q. **Are there support groups for women who suffer from PMS?**

A. There are PMS support groups throughout the country. I encourage you to find one. It should promote ideas that assist people in getting well.

Some support groups (not just PMS groups) fail to provide positive guidelines and ideas for recovery. In a group with positive guidelines, healthy, constructive ideas and attitudes can develop. Women who share the same problem find it comforting to know that they are not alone in their situation.

Q. I'm lucky to have a husband who believes in and understands my PMS. But it has been a struggle to get a professional to listen to me. A few gynecologists have told me they don't really believe in PMS. Because of the symptoms, I began to wonder if it is all in my head. I've known for some time this was something I couldn't control without help. Through friends, I found a doctor who has put me on the right track: proper diet, vitamins and medical treatment. I know I'm not cured, but I can now take charge of my life. My symptoms are not entirely gone, but because I now understand them and am in treatment, I can keep my problems under control. No longer is everything a crisis.

I'd like some information on starting a PMS support group. I want to help others understand that they are not alone and that there is help for them.

A. It is nice to hear from someone who has experienced success in getting her PMS symptoms under control. It sounds as if your support system has been effective and that you have worked hard to find a satisfactory solution.

Why not contact the doctor who assisted you

in your quest for a solution and let her know of your interest in helping other women with PMS? She may have several other PMS patients who have requested more information about the syndrome. She could put you in touch with some of them. If you are unsuccessful taking this approach, you could contact the hospital or university medical school in the closest large city. The obstetrics and gynecologoy department may have names of women who have expressed an interest and are just waiting for others to form a group. Also, I would suggest you contact your local mental health practitioners.

Q. Besides the medical communitiy, is there support for women with PMS?

A. In some situations, you can find support groups that are not connected to the medical community. Some of these groups are created informally by women who have PMS, and others are available through the mental health community.

Q. You have mentioned PMS Access. What is it, and how can I get in touch with this group? Do they give support group referrals?

A. *PMS Access* is an organization in Madison, Wisconsin which specializes in providing women with information and products to deal with PMS. Their number is 1 800-558-7046. They also are a referral source and may have some suggestions for support groups in your area.

Q. **How do you form a support group that helps everyone?**

A. There are many qualities that a good support group will have. A facilitator who is familiar with PMS is one of the key ingredients. It is also important to have a regular meeting time and place. Stay away from groups where "misery loves company" is the theme. You don't want to get together to simply complain! You want to do something about your PMS—a positive message coming from the group experience is essential. You can encourage each other's recovery by sharing ideas on diet and exercise and other measures that have helped alleviate your symptoms.

Q. **I am not a medical person, but I suffer with PMS and lead a support group. How do I keep the group interesting and keep women coming every week?**

A. Why not organize a group to meet for a specified amount of time, such as six consecutive weeks? Pick a subject for each week that would be of interest, such as PMS in the workplace, PMS and parenting or PMS and men. You might also ask someone who speaks on the topic of PMS to be a guest one night. Let the prospective participants know how important their attendance is for the continuity of the group. Addressing these areas would create more consistant participation.

Q. **Many women, like myself, have made concerted efforts to organize and direct self-help** groups for women suffering from varying degrees of PMS distress. In consulting with other organizers, I do find that it is difficult to sustain the membership of such a group. Yet women congregate in halls and hospital offices in great numbers to listen to specialists, doctors and authorities paid to speak. There, they are exposed to many of the same ideas they would encounter in any good group. Do you think this suggests a dependency on the professional answer versus the work of a self-help group?

A. Your observations are interesting, but I don't think the answer is quite so simple. Information from authorities on any given subject serves a different purpose than the support that is received from a self-help group. Because the field of PMS is relatively young, new data is likely to come from the professionals studying the subject. It makes sense that women's interest would be high in seeking this input. Yet this type of information gathering cannot provide the same kind of support as a self-help group. I have also found that PMS self-help groups are hard to maintain for long periods of time. It may be better to organize a PMS group that meets for six to eight weeks and then disbands with the idea that another group would be organized after a two to three week break if enough interest is indicated.

Q. My husband and family members need a support group to help them cope with my PMS. The ups and downs are so extreme day-to-day that they never know how I really feel or

**what to expect from me. I have tried every-
thing to help them understand.**

A. I agree with you. Family members need to
share information with other people who are experiencing the same problems. While I know that
direct conversations with your family is essential, I
also think that support groups for family members
similar to Al Anon are an excellent idea.

Q. **I think my wife has PMS but is unaware of
it. What can I do?**

A. Develop your sense of timing and educate
yourself. You need to let your wife know what you
are thinking. She may or may not receive this
information willingly. Approach the subject during
her symptom-free time when she is less likely to be
defensive. Thoroughly educate yourself about
PMS so that when you broach the subject, you
know what you are talking about. No one wants to
be told that there is something wrong with them.
Be sensitive, non-accusational and supportive in
delivering your information.

Q. **I'm fairly sure that I have identified PMS in
my wife. How and when do I decide to discuss
this with her for the most favorable results?**

A. Your question is the one most frequently
asked by husbands and significant others. Men
are reluctant to bring up the subject of PMS when
their partners are irritable and depressed because
of being premenstrual. On the other hand, they
also hesitate to discuss PMS during the good time

of the month because they don't want to spoil the positive time. Yet in view of the two choices, it's still a better idea to open the topic of PMS during your wife's symptom-free time of the month.

Q. As a man living with a woman who has PMS, what can I do to help?

A. Educate yourself! Look at PMS as a medical condition that you can deal with effectively. Offer your support to your friend. Just by helping her identify PMS you are demonstrating your willingness to work with her. Become part of an effective support system for her. Let her know that you are willing to go the extra mile for her while she is getting PMS under control. That could involve anything from helping out with the chores at home to allowing her some extra space during her premenstrual time. Take heart in the fact that the identification and treatment of PMS goes on for a finite period of time. You probably will not be called on to do the extras for very long.

Q. What should I do to prevent my rages during my PMS days?

A. Do not engage! If you detect that today is a no win day, try not to become involved in arguments or disagreements with the PMS woman. This may be easier said than done. It is important to resist the temptation to enter into a discussion which could lead to a disagreement. Verbalize that you do not want to discuss the subject at this time or choose the non-verbal route of getting some space, even if that means taking a two to three minute break and leaving the room. By separating yourself even momentarily, you interrupt the tension and avoid risking loss of control.

Q. **Has a book been published to help husbands or children have a better understanding of PMS?**

A. Yes. My first book, *PMS: A Positive Program To Gain Control* addresses, among other topics, the concerns of children and spouses as they relate to PMS.

Q. **What can my wife and I do to explain PMS to our eight- and eleven-year-olds? My wife is just now getting help, but the kids are still very confused about Mom's recent ups and downs.**

A. Children are all too willing to take on responsibility for problems in the family which really have very little to do with them. Talk to your children in terms that they can understand. Start the conversation by stating that you have something very important to talk about. It is a good idea for Mom to begin by telling them that she has a physical imbalance which is present in her body during part of the month. Be sure to mention that she is going to look the same to them while the imbalance is present; however, she may not act the same. By telling them that she may have a shorter temper and may not be as involved with them during her imbalanced time, Mom takes responsibility for her behavior instead of the children wondering what they did wrong to make her so angry or distant.

Q. What are five ways I can help my wife deal with PMS?

A. These suggestions are taken from *PMS: A Positive Program To Gain Control* (The Body Press, 1988):

- Create healthy diversions. If she is upset, ask her to go for a walk with you. If she is tired from caring for the kids, step in and take over.
- Demonstrate support for her by reading the literature on PMS or accompanying her to a PMS clinic. Your interest and presence tell her that you care and want to be supportive.
- Tell her that you appreciate what she is going through and that you support her.
- Be sensitive to the situation by focusing on what needs to be done. Don't wait for her to ask. If the kids need to eat, feed them.
- Cultivate lots of patience.

Resources
for Information
About PMS

BIBLIOGRAPHY

MEDICAL TREATMENTS AND PMS
> Hufnagel, Vicki, G., M.D. with Susan K. Golant. *No More Hysterectomies*. New American Library, New York, 1988.

WHAT CAN I DO TO HELP MYSELF
> Morgan Stewart with contributions from Dr. Allen Stewart and Dr. Guy Abraham. *Beat PMS Through Diet*. Ebury Press, London, 1987.

MEDICAL ARTICLES ABOUT PMS

CAUSES OF PMS
> Katharina Dalton, M.D. *The Premenstrual Syndrome and Progesterone Therapy*, Second Edition, Year Book Medical Publishers, Inc., Chicago, Illinois, 1984.

> R.L. Reid, M.D. and S.C.C. Yen, M.D., "Premenstrual Syndrome," *American Journal of Obstetrics and Gynecology*, Vol. 139, No. 1, 1981, pp. 85-104.

David R. Rubinow, M.D., and Peter Roy-Burne, M.D., "Premenstrual Syndromes: Overview from a Methodologic Perspective," *American Journal of Psychiatry*, Vol. 141, No. 2, February 1984, pp. 163-172.

PMS AND MENSTRUAL CRAMPS

John F. Steege, M.D., Anna L. Stout, Ph.D., and Sharon L. Rupp, R.N.C., "Relationships Among Premenstrual Symptoms and Menstrual Cycle Characteristics," *Obstetrics and Gynecology*, Vol. 65, No. 3, March 1985, pp. 398-402.

Penny W. Budoff, M.D., *No More Menstrual Cramps and Other Good News*, Penguin, New York, 1980.

PMS AND PSYCHIATRIC ILLNESS

Renate DeJong, Ph.D., David R. Rubinow, M.D., Peter Roy-Byrne, M.D., Christine Hoban, M.S.W., Gay N. Grover, M.S.N., and Robert M. Post, M.D., "Premenstrual Mood Disorder and Psychiatric Illness," *American Journal of Psychiatry*, Vol. 142, No. 11, November 1985, pp. 1359-1361.

David R. Rubinow, M.D., Christine Hoban, M.S.W., Peter Roy-Byrne, M.D., Gay N. Grover, M.S.N., and Robert M. Post, M.D., "Premenstrual Syndromes: Past and Future Research Strategies," *Canadian Journal of Psychiatry*, Vol. 30, November 1985, pp. 469-473.

PMS AND PSYCHOLOGICAL ASSESSMENT

Anna L. Stout, Ph.D., and John F. Steege, M.D., "Psychological Assessment of

Women Seeking Treatment for Pre-menstrual Syndrome," *Journal of Psychosomatic Research*, Vol. 29, No. 6, 1985, pp. 621-629.

PMS AND PROGESTERONE

Katharina Dalton, M.D., *The Premenstrual Syndrome and Progesterone Therapy*, Second Edition, Year Book Medical Publishers, Inc., Chicago, Illinois, 1984.

Ronald V. Norris, M.D., "Progesterone for Premenstrual Tension," *Journal of Reproductive Medicine*, Vol. 28, No. 8, August 1983. pp. 509-516.

PHARMACOLOGICAL ADVICE

Madison Pharmacy Associates
429 Gammon Place
Madison, Wisconsin 53719
1-800-558-7046

INFORMATION, COUNSELING AND PRESENTATIONS

PreMenstrual Syndrome Clinic
2760 29th Street, Suite 205
Boulder, Colorado 80301
303-440-7100

PMS NEWSLETTER

PMS Access
P.O. Box 9326
Madison, Wisconsin 53715
1-800-222-4PMS

INDEX